Quantum Weight Loss 4 Life

By John Luckey

I0410504

Contents

Introduction

You are what you eat, right? So toss out all those fad diets and eat healthy! But you want to lose weight, you say. Again I say, toss out the fad diets and eat healthy and you will not only lose weight, you will keep it off and live long and prosper. Well, at least I can assure you that will you be around longer to enjoy your new body. Fad diets may offer some immediate weight loss and a temporary figure in the mirror that you like better, but they will also wear you out before your time and before you know it you will be swimming through the sea of life like a porpoise, bobbing and weaving up and down—fat, then skinny, then fat, then skinny, and never truly healthy.

I am going to show you how you can have it all. Be healthy, eat healthy, and have that fit athletic body you know you want to see in the mirror. The truth is that diets—the wrong foods in the wrong amounts—are killing you.

A recent news program quoted a study that claims many of us go to sleep at night worried that a meteor will strike the planet or climate change will spin us out of control or that a terrorist attack or something out of our control will kill us. I have good news: that's statistically unlikely. The bad news is you're killing yourself with your lifestyle. Not only is much of the world becoming overweight, but many are taking harmful drugs to deal with the diseases caused by the obesity that they brought on themselves. It is time to stop the craziness and break the cycle.

Weight-loss-4-life fact: The average American woman now weighs 166. 2 pounds, about the same as the average American man weighed in the early 1960s. Over the same time, U.S. men have gained nearly 30 pounds, from 166.3 in the 60s to 195.5 today. Can you say "save the whales"? No offense to Shamu, but we are becoming whales. We need a quantum lifestyle change and we need it now. Not a passing fad, but true weight loss 4 life, a healthy lifestyle change that will reshape our lives so we like the person in the mirror. Real weight loss 4 life incorporated into a healthy lifestyle change might just save our lives as well.

So why don't fad diets work? Clearly, they must have some value or people would not chase after them, one diet after another.

Have you ever watched Usain Bolt run the 100 meters or the 200 meter race in the Olympics? Have you noticed there isn't an ounce of fat on him? We'll come back to that in a minute. When Mr. Bolt prepares to run the 100 meter dash, he crouches down, and gets into the blocks. When the starter's pistol is fired, he explodes out of the blocks with short fast strides, then quickly shifts into a long stride that he maintains throughout the race, with grace.

Fad diets are the starting blocks in this race… at best. They are not meant to be sustained throughout the race. You need to shift gears and catch your stride for life. A sound diet might be helpful in starting the race, much as the starting blocks assist a sprinter at the beginning of his race. Have you ever seen a sprinter carry his starting blocks with him throughout the race? No, me either. They are designed to assist you at the beginning of the race and become terribly dysfunctional if you carry them with you throughout the race. It's the same thing with a diet.

Weight loss 4 life is a lifestyle change. It doesn't mean you're signing up for basic training or that you're going to get stuck with K rations for the rest of your life or ordering your meals from a distributor that you saw on TV for the next ten years.

The lifestyle change I'm going to share with

you in this book will be easy to understand, fun, effective, and sustainable. Some of you are ready to go right now, but others just got stuck on the word "change." Please don't be intimidated by a small word like change. I'm certain you've heard the old saying, "The definition of insanity is doing the same thing repeatedly and expecting different results," and clearly something deep inside of you is desiring change or you would not have read this far and I honor that.

Consider this: today your bank account sits at zero. Tomorrow you find you've won the lottery and instantly your bank account has changed for the better. That wasn't hard, was it?

This book is that kind of change. Let's go. Mr. Bolt is waiting!

Chapter 1: The Facts You Need

In a perfect world, your perfect weight is a simple function of your calories consumed versus the calories you burn. Period. Yes, pretty much like the engine in your car. Simple math, but in case you have not noticed, this is not a perfect world. There are other issues involved in finding your ideal weight. At one point in your life you may have functioned as a simple math equation—calories in, calories out—no sweat, your engine ran smoothly. However, dysfunction is a reality in an imperfect world so any functional long-term solution to a problem, any problem (in this case, your weight) must deal with all of the facts in your ever-changing reality.

True weight loss 4 life must consider many variables. We will start with simple math, yes, but if that is not working, then we will find out why and correct the dysfunctions so the equation works again. For instance, if you are obese, low on energy, lethargic, can't get started in the morning, check your body temperature for a few days before you get out of bed. If it is 97.6 or below, it would be wise to consult your physician and have your thyroid checked. If your thyroid is not functioning ideally, it can mess up your math... so to speak.

I know a lot of you are saying, "Math? I hated that class in high school. I thought I was done with that!" Well, relax, you are not a math equation but your physical body does operate according to math and quantum physics. Don't worry, you won't need a PhD to lose and maintain your ideal weight. It really doesn't have to be that complex.

A deeper understanding shows us that there is more than simple math and higher quantum physics that make you tick. You are a mind-body-spirit matrix: MBSM, as I call it. You're a complex person. You always knew that, right? So, how do we keep the understanding of this complexity simple? We break it down into bite-size pieces, of course. Please, don't let that little word *math* intimidate you any more than the word *change* did. Remember our example? Your bank account is empty today and tomorrow you win the lottery; that's change and that's math and that's good, right?

The math is simple and it always works, but sometimes it is distorted by environmental factors, such as emotional, financial, and physical stress, chemical and hormonal imbalances, and metabolic factors. We will address the distortions that these factors cause and you will be able to reestablish a functional simple math operating system. This is where many weight loss systems fail. Some may work for a while—forcing the math to work temporarily—but if the underlying dysfunction is not identified and addressed, there will be a relapse and a subsequent regain of weight that is often greater than the original condition.

Weight loss 4 life is a comprehensive mind-body-spirit approach designed to identify the dysfunctions and then allow you to correct them in all areas of your life, so that your lifelong solution becomes simple again! Are you ready?

Let's take an incredible journey within your body and learn how your vital systems operate. Again, don't worry; we are not looking to get a PhD, just some understanding. I promise to keep it simple and focus on a functional understanding of how we operate. Why? Well, if somebody gives you keys to the space shuttle and allows you to sit inside, it still won't go anywhere unless you know how to operate it, right? I know the space shuttle's been retired for some time, but you're not, so let's get going!

I mentioned earlier that you are like an engine... fuel in and fuel burned and exhaust out. The key is if you want to lose weight, burn more fuel then you take in. If you are a simple one fuel source engine your vehicle—you—will soon end up stalled beside the road. That's what happens when you burn more fuel than you take in; you run out of gas. But remember when I said you're complex? Well, you really are; in fact, you have a hybrid engine and you can burn several different types of fuel. Your engine can burn carbohydrates, and it can burn fat, and it can burn protein.

Your two main fuel sources are carbohydrates and fat. Protein is your reserve tank. If you are burning from that reserve tank you're tearing down your muscles and that's not good. In fact, your muscles are also your main engine! They burn the most fuel, so the more muscles you have, the more fuel you burn and the more food you can eat. That's why a professional bodybuilder who weighs 300 pounds doesn't have an ounce of fat on him and yet can still eat more in a day than your family budgets for the next month; big engines need much fuel. Most bodybuilders understand more about nutrition than most dietitians or physicians ever will. It is not just steroids and heavy weights that cause them to look like Greek gods; it's also knowledge of how their engines work. Not only are you equipped with large hybrid engines that can burn multiple fuels, but believe it or not, every cell in your body has a small engine within it, called the mitochondria. But wait a minute, I promised you wouldn't have to have a PhD, so we'll stay with the big concepts, the big engines, for now.

Bodybuilders know how much of each of the different fuel sources their engines need. They also know which exercises and which levels of intensity burn the different fuels. I will share more of that with you later, but for now I want you to remember the fundamentals.

Let's talk about total calorie balance, that simple math equation that when all other dysfunctions are corrected determines whether you gain weight or lose weight or remain steady at your current weight. The good news is you don't have to run all day like a marathon runner to lose weight. Believe it or not, even in idle your engine is burning 50 to 70 percent of the calories needed to balance that equation. Physicians and exercise physiologists call that the resting energy expenditure (REE) or Basal Metabolic Rate (BMR). This is the rate at which your body burns calories for basic bodily functions, such as, well, general housekeeping like breathing, manufacturing cells, and maintaining body temperature. In other words, if you woke up but never got out of bed all day, you would still burn 50 to 70 percent of the calories needed to maintain your normal weight with your present caloric intake. That's the good news.

Hopefully, though, you can see from this example that if you indeed did not get out of bed and still maintained your present diet, you would be gaining weight because you're burning only a maximum of 70 percent of the calories you're eating. If you got out of bed and went about your daily chores maintaining your normal caloric intake, you would maintain your current weight. If you got out of bed and went about your daily chores and added a common sense exercise routine and maintained your current caloric intake, you would begin to lose weight. It's just that simple.

You may have guessed it by now, but the person more likely to burn 70 percent of his or her normal daily caloric intake at rest is the one with the biggest engines: the bodybuilder. Those big muscles or big engines are going to burn more calories even doing nothing. Those with small muscles, whether they have a lot of fat or not, are more likely to be on the 50 percent end of the scale for a Basal Metabolic Rate (BMR). The moral of the story this far is that if you want to be efficient at losing weight you want to have an efficient engine that burns lots of calories, even when it's idling. In other words, incorporate resistance exercises into your life and build more muscle. Don't worry, you don't have to build as much muscle as Arnold did to see a difference.

In addition to your body composition, your age, genes, and gender largely determine your BMR, which means much of your energy use is predetermined. However, you can alter that by altering your body composition. You can change your BMR! One way you can also alter your BMR and body composition is by determining how much and what type of exercise you get each day.

Clearly the foundation in the kingdom of body shaping is BMR. It is the starting place for everything else. It's the baseline, hence the term basal metabolic rate. Once you have your BMR you can begin to create a lifestyle that is healthy and allows you to shape your body the way you want it without crazy crash diets. So how do you figure BMR? I'm glad you asked!

Well, short of measuring it in a clinical environment, there is the Mifflin-St. Jeor equation, a formula introduced in 1990. The Mifflin-St. Jeor equation is now considered the standard when it comes to calculating BMR. Here is how it works:

Mifflin-St. Jeor Equation

For men: BMR = 10 x weight (kg) + 6.25 x height (cm) – 5 x age (years) + 5

For women: BMR = 10 x weight (kg) + 6.25 x height (cm) – 5 x age (years) – 161

(1 inch is equal to 2.45 cm and 1lbs is equal to 0.45359237 kilogram)

While not perfect (and that's a subject for Chapter 5: "What's eating you"), the BMR is a great place to start. Once you have your BMR, you can add your estimates of your caloric burn rate from your exercise programs, and determine a comfortable and balanced caloric intake that meets your goals.

Wait a minute, I hear someone saying, balanced caloric intake? What is this… more math? The answer is simple, yes, and the math is simple, too; in fact, there are a lot of great apps for smart phones nowadays, such as "my fitness pal" that will do all the work for you.

Of course, if you're eating at home and out of a package, it will list how many calories per serving and the serving size, etc. There are also sites on the Internet that will list the caloric content of nearly any food you can think of. But if you have a smart phone, it might be a smart choice to pick up one of those smart apps! Good news—many are for free, and they will do all the work for you.

Now you know what you need to do. The math is simple and the smart phone apps are incredible, and the bottom line will become obvious. You are burning X amount of calories. You want to lose weight in a reasonable manner. Therefore until you reach that goal, you will consume X minus Y calories per day until your ultimate weight goals are reached. You choose the value for Y based on how fast you want to lose the weight. Perhaps a few hundred calories less a day. Small steps are something I can handle; by staying active I don't miss the few calories. But put me in front of a TV for hours and I get lazy and want chips and salsa and Haagen-Dazs.

Speaking of staying active, if you do some

interval, or strength, or cardio training, you will, of course, burn a few more calories than your current BMR. That is in your favor, too! I lost twenty-two pounds in twenty days doing just that! I moved—literally! In the process I unconsciously reduced my calorie intake, because I was too busy packing and unpacking, loading and unloading etc., to eat large portions and sit around waiting for it to digest! Moving is a very tedious interval training program that I don't recommend unless you have to, but it does burn fat! When I finally got most of my things unpacked I simply recalculated my BMR and my allotted daily caloric intake to maintain that weight, and built a balanced healthy lifestyle and diet around those figures. I guarantee if you do that (not the house move, but some movement) you're going to like your figure, and you will be healthier than you've ever been before. A fit body boot camp class is more fun than moving… just saying, or perhaps you would like to lift some weights. I do and love it! It is my meditation time in the gym, where I can forget everything else! It's good mind-body-spirit time.

Above all, It's important to reject a diet mentality. If you adopt restrictive negative thinking you are going to feel deprived and ultimately defeated, and this will most likely trigger over eating and possibly even the development of an eating disorder. To reach your healthy weight, don't diet, but rather, eat healthy and move your body to adjust your caloric burn rate using the tools above, with intake portion control. When you reach your desired goal, do the simple math and maintain your desired goal. See, you didn't need a PhD to change your life after all.

Let me ask you a question. When you lose that weight you want to lose, where does it go? I don't mean from your waist to your belly, etc. I mean when you have lost that 10, 20, or even 100 pounds you want to lose …where does it go? Quantum physicists probably have some answers already because they know that matter is never really destroyed, it's just re-formed. Fat is matter, so where does it go? How does it leave your body?

I hear some asking, "What does it matter? If it leaves, I don't care where it goes… Just keep going."

Well, I'll tell you why it matters. Billions are spent each year by naïve consumers looking for the next magic pill that will melt fat away right before their eyes in the mirror without doing a thing. That's making con artists rich and keeping you fat.

Here are the facts. Fairy dust doesn't burn fat, but math and quantum physics do, so if you want to master your figure, forget the fairy tales and embrace the mystery of you and how you work.

You are 70-90 percent water, depending on the expert you choose to believe. I am sure you all know the chemical "alias" (formula) for water: H_2O. That's two hydrogen atoms and one oxygen atom in the water molecule.

So what is the chemical formula or alias for human fat? $C55H104O6$. An average fat molecule has 55 carbon atoms, 104 hydrogen atoms (sometimes more or less, depending on the type of fat), and always just 6 oxygen atoms. A bit larger than water, right? The difference between what I looked like and the sizably larger pants I wore before my move was this molecule; well, not just one, an entire clan of them, I think. Remember, I dropped twenty-two pounds in twenty days and "skinnied up" enough to go from a 39-inch waist to a 34 during that time. Some of those clothes I moved I didn't have to bring! I was happy the pounds were gone, but where did they go? I figured I needed to know so that I could guard the gate and not let them back in; you get my point? Most people who lose weight without knowing what they are doing will gain it and more back before too long, much like many lotto winners who win the lottery and then end up broke again within three years.

To prevent a relapse, are you willing to look with me just for a minute at the math of getting the fat out?

You know that for a fire to burn you need oxygen, right? Well, the same is true of fat. Your body must supply oxygen to burn those fat molecules and the result of that reaction in your cells is $55CO_2$ plus 52 H_2Os. In other words, you break the fat down to carbon dioxide and water! Carbon dioxide? Yep, that's right; stay fat or contribute to climate change. Sorry, that excuse won't fly. Seriously, those who have had a rudimentary understanding of how we work know that we breathe in oxygen and breathe out carbon dioxide, which the plants and trees use to convert back into oxygen for us. They need our CO_2 to live! So clearly not all CO_2 is bad; without it we are history and so are the plants and trees. Good try, though.

What am I saying? When you burn fat you

produce water and CO_2. The CO_2 is expelled in your breath where nature starts turning it back into O_2 and the water is disposed of as urine, feces, and sweat. You need O_2 to burn the fat and CO_2 and H_2O to carry the fat residue away… far, far away. So in finding out where it goes, you also found out how it works. It's not magic, it's science, and since it is science, it can be measured and understood.

You already learned that 50 to 70 percent of your caloric intake is burned just running this great system nature has provided. If you step on the accelerator a bit on a regular basis, daily, you will raise your burn rate and consume more O_2 and burn more fat… and all things being the same, you will lose weight. If you decrease your intake of new fuel and all other factors remain the same, you will switch to the alternative fuel of fat and you will lose weight.

You see, there are two places in the equation where you can influence the result. You can raise your physical activity and your caloric burn rate above the fuel supply on hand and cause your body to switch to a reserve fuel. That's number one. Number two, you can decrease your intake and switch to the alternative fuel and burn and "dispose of the adipose." In lieu of a three-year course in quantum physics, math, and biochemistry remember this: eat less and move more.

The most successful lifelong transitions to a healthy lifestyle and ideal weight involve balancing both of those variables. Remember, you are a hybrid vehicle and you can burn multiple fuels. The key is having just enough in the reserve tank. You don't need, or want, to tow a trailer behind you with a huge reserve tank that is slowing you down and creating excessive wear and tear on your system! There are plenty of fueling stations on our journey of life, so there really is no need to store up like Jabba the Hutt. Clearly, most of us do not set out to do so. Life happens and distractions occur that interrupt our fat burning sessions and then we sit down and eat too much to soothe the guilt we have for not caring for our bodies with exercise (our fat burning sessions) and before you know it...

Life will always offer us a choice. We can let the distractions and emergencies of life get us off track and accept the consequences, or stay on course in a balanced mature manner, understanding that there will always be unknowns and distractions, but we do not have to allow them power over us. Go for a walk on a nature trail, go to the gym and make it your meditation time to balance your mind, body, and spirit. It is your sacred privilege. It is your sacred duty. Call it temple maintenance and look forward to it with your entire being. Each time you do, you will reap great dividends in every dimension.

Chapter 2: What About a Jump Start?

In years past we burned almost as many calories as we ate just preparing our food. Even if you were a well off professional you were most likely a land owner, a gentleman farmer, and grew your own food. Even if you didn't plow the fields yourself, you moved about the fields as you watched over and managed the operation. If you were a member of the poorer class, you burned even more calories as you stalked prey and hunted for your food.

Now we sit at work and sit at recreation watching TV, playing video games, etc. Often we don't move our burn rate much above our resting BMR! The microwave is burning the calories in our modern kitchens now; what used to take hours on our feet now takes minutes in a chair waiting for the microwave to work its magic. It warms our food in seconds and over time turns us into marshmallows. When we finally stop and look in the mirror and see the damage, we want it fixed instantly as well. Bad news, it just doesn't work that way.

Good news, it is never too late to get up and get back in the race. Speaking of that—the race, that is—remember Mr. Bolt, the fastest man alive? Even he uses a jump start at the beginning of his race. He crouches down and explodes out of the starting blocks at the sound of the starter's pistol. But that is a fraction of the race; yes, it is a jump start and gets him up to speed faster, and in this world we all want that. The key here is to realize that a jump start is just that: a start. It will not serve you well into the race of life. It is a tool for short term use.

In the beginning of your journey back to your ideal self you may indeed "eat less" as well as "move more," and when you reach your desired goal you may only "move more." That is one type of jump start. Others are available as well, under the care of a physician. My wife, a physician, assists many patients in a safe and sane approach to temporarily boost their metabolic rate, getting them out of the blocks in the race back to their ideal selves. The key words here are *safe* and *sane* usage and for a *limited* period of time. It is used as a jump start, not a lifestyle change, and that is really what you want, a lifestyle change that will improve your health and well being as well as your image in the mirror for life. The focus of this book is lifestyle change that leads to a sustainable new you. In the process I want to share with you an overview of all the options that you have available to you short term and long term. Physician prescribed and monitored pharmaceuticals are a short term legitimate jump start for some patients.

While you are at your physician's office, make sure to have them evaluate your hormones as well. As I mentioned earlier, hormonal imbalance is one thing that can take the simple math of weight loss and weight management and make it complex. You really want to make certain that your doctor has a good understanding of endocrinology, the science of hormones and how they make you tick, because they are interrelated and complex.

Think of them as the mobile that hangs over a baby's crib. There are many figures suspended and rotating from the motor above. If you touch one of them and alter its course around the circle... it affects the direction of all of them. So it is with hormones; they are a tightly knit bunch that stick together and what affects one can have a counter affect on another.

This is not an endocrinology textbook and I am not going to turn it into one (as much fun as that would be for me). However, I will give you a few examples of how important it is to have them working with you, not against you. After all, you want a jump start, not an anchor to the past to drag behind you!

I mentioned that if your body temperature is below normal each morning before arising you should have your thyroid hormone levels checked. Your thyroid hormone is the regulator for your metabolism in every cell of your body and clearly, if it is deficient, you will not be burning the calories you were designed to burn and the result will be weight gain. Yes, sometimes even if you eat less and move more! You see how important it is?

Here is how the plot thickens with hormones. If you are under a lot of stress (and who isn't these days), it is possible that your "stress hormones" are suppressing your thyroid and messing up your simple math equation at several levels. If your sustained stress is producing excessive stress hormones that are suppressing your thyroid, then your cells have their thermostats turned way down, so they are not burning calories as they should be.

So how can we melt fat away fast with hormones? By making certain they are balanced and working as designed! One way that is done is with moderate regular interval training exercise. It helps normalize your thyroid. It helps counteract stress and it releases good hormones and endorphins, etc., into your system that will counteract the emotional and physical effects of stress.

Most of us have no idea that our hormones are controlling everything! Every dimension of our ability to lose weight is governed by hormones, how our bodies respond to our food intake (diet), where we store our fat, our appetite, our cravings. It's all controlled by hormones. And you thought you were in control! Keep reading and you will be very soon.

Let's start with a quick look at what your thyroid does for you. Your thyroid is one of the largest endocrine glands and greatly influences almost every cell in your body. It regulates your metabolism and controls your weight, because it is intimately involved in the fat burning process throughout each cell of your body. Thyroid hormones are also required for the growth and development in children and in nearly every process in your body. When your thyroid levels are out of balance, so are you. Too much or too little hormone secretion from this gland can create trouble for your overall health and well-being. It can make you too hot, too cold, too lethargic, too wired and a host of other symptoms. I've read studies that indicate that between 10 and 40 percent of the people living in the United States have sub optimal thyroid function. Low thyroid function has been linked to serious health conditions like fibromyalgia, irritable bowel syndrome, acne, eczema, gum disease, infertility, and many autoimmune diseases.

The thyroid is a butterfly shaped gland about two inches wide that sits right by your vocal cords. It produces three types of hormones that doctors call T3 and T4 and T2. These hormones from the thyroid interact with all of your hormones, including insulin, cortisol, and sex hormones like estrogen and progesterone and testosterone. The fact is that these hormones are all intimately tied together and are in constant communication with each other. Perhaps now you can begin to see that a low thyroid or a high thyroid hormone count can affect everything else in your body. That's why when your thyroid output is low there are so many widespread symptoms and diseases that it can cause.

Let's look at a percentage breakdown of the thyroid hormones. 90 percent of thyroid hormones are produced in the form of T4. It is an inactive form of thyroid. Your liver—when needed—converts T4 into T3, the active form, with the help of an enzyme. T2 is currently the least understood component of the thyroid function, so for now T3 is the hormone we are most concerned with. If everything is working properly, you will make what you need and have the correct amount of T3 and T4, which literally controls the metabolism of every cell in your body. If your T3 is low either by scarce production or not converting properly from T4, your entire system suffers.

The T3 hormone is critically important. It tells the nucleus of your cells to send messages to your DNA to speed up your metabolism by burning fat. When found in the proper amounts T3 usually lowers cholesterol levels, regrows hair, and keeps you lean. It is important to realize that your T3 levels can be affected by a number of sources. Your all-important T3 levels can be disrupted by stress, environmental toxins, allergens, infections, and nutritional imbalances. These can lead to complications including hyperthyroidism or hypothyroidism, and even cancer in some cases.

The hormonal or endocrine system is interrelated and very complex, much like a three-dimensional chess board. If you have a problem and you believe it involves your hormones, it is imperative that you get a good physician as your coach.

For the purpose of this book I'm going to take a moment and go over some of the symptoms of hypothyroidism, or underactive thyroid. Identifying hypothyroidism purely from symptoms can be a bit hard to do since symptoms may overlap with other diseases. In the past hypothyroidism was often missed as some clues went undetected using only traditional tests to check thyroid levels, so again, make sure your physician either has a good understanding of endocrinology or refers you to an endocrinologist who will order all the correct tests.

Typically, an underactive thyroid leaves you lethargic and fatigued with a lack of energy. Sometimes depression is linked to the condition. If you have not had a good night's sleep in the last week and you are burning the candle at both ends, you're tired and you have a lack of energy, resist the urge to blame your thyroid and get a good night's sleep first. When you've done that and you still suffer from fatigue and cannot sustain energy long enough compared with past levels of fitness or abilities, it may be time to test your thyroid function.

If your thyroid foundation is weak, sustaining energy is going to be a challenge. You will notice that you just don't seem to have the energy like you used to have. If you have an unexplained weight gain or difficulty losing weight—despite an aggressive exercise program and careful eating—you might have hypothyroidism. If your skin is dry and coarse and your hair is tangled and dry, and if you seem to have perpetually dry skin that doesn't respond well to most moisturizing lotions or creams, you might have hypothyroidism. If you have an unexplained hair loss, especially women, you might have hypothyroidism. If you seem to feel cold all the time even when others don't, you might have hypothyroidism, and as we mentioned earlier, if you're resting body temperature is less than 97.6 it may be an indication of hypothyroidism.

Please don't become a hypochondriac like many in this internet generation. We all know someone who has read about a disease and its symptoms and is convinced he or she has it and is going to die because of it. On the other hand, it can be very helpful to your physician to have accurate facts and symptoms to share when looking for the cause of unexplained weight gain.

So, while you wait to see an endocrinologist or your test results, remain calm and just stick to the facts. What can you do in the meantime to improve your thyroid health? The experts suggest avoiding environmental toxins such as bromine and other halogens. Make sure you have a diet that includes iodine rich foods. Make certain you're getting adequate rest. And finally, minimize your stress levels by taking some breaks in your busy day to meditate, daydream, or if you can, soak in a hot tub. Your health and your productivity will improve if you take time to "go on a vacation" in your mind several times throughout the day.

I find meditating to the sound of Centerpoint's Holosync® technology extremely relaxing with a number of positive side effects, such as laying down new neural pathways between the left and right hemispheres of the brain and enhancing great sleep. During those deep sleep cycles Growth Hormone is released that does many good things for your body, mind, and spirit!

One more very important thing I'll bet you thought I forgot. Exercise! For me exercise is my primary form of meditation. It's mind-body-spirit balancing time and I look forward to it every day. What does exercise do for your thyroid gland? Exercise directly stimulates your thyroid to secrete more thyroid hormone and increases the sensitivity of all your tissues to that thyroid hormone. It is thought by some experts that many of the health benefits of exercise stem directly from improved thyroid function. So, go for a morning walk, have a lunchtime workout, or an evening swim. Whatever it is that works for you, let your imagination go and find fun ways to exercise because you are losing weight and healing yourself in the process.

In our look at hormones and how they affect our weight loss and weight gain I chose to consider the thyroid first because of its importance to all the other hormones. When your thyroid is in balance the math works, and when you're taking that walk or playing a game of tennis you're melting those pounds away without even thinking about it. On the other hand, if you're not getting enough sleep because you're worried about your weight and then you begin to restrict your caloric intake because you're worried about your weight, guess what? You're going to increase your cortisol—the stress hormone—which is going to suppress your thyroid and send out signals to all the cells in your body to slow down and not burn so much fuel. Even if you go to the gym because you're so stressed out about it all, you may still gain weight. I suggest you educate yourself so that you understand how hormones can "mess up your math" and then relax and relieve the stress; have fun with your exercise and have fun with the new healthy dietary ideas you will learn here. Get your hormones balanced and watch how your life becomes balanced as well. Then enjoy the new you that appears in the mirror.

Of course there are other hormones that affect weight gain and weight loss. Another major player is insulin, so let's look at it next.

A word of caution. If you remain reluctant to dig in and learn what you need to know about hormones, if you are still asking, "Why do we need to know about all these hormones?" I have one short answer for you. It is because any form of hormonal imbalance will sabotage your efforts at weight loss, regardless of your diet and exercise habits. It's not complicated, but it is important!

You can get everything else right and not make good progress in weight control if you allow your insulin levels to get out of whack. Insulin is an essential hormone whose main function is to process sugar in the bloodstream and carry it into the cells where it is used as fuel or stored as fat. Insulin levels that are constantly high will prevent you from burning the fat you have stored and that you now want to use for fuel. It is virtually impossible to have high levels of insulin in your system while burning fat at the same time. Think about that for a moment.

Insulin is a hormone that causes most of the body's cells to absorb glucose from the blood for fuel. In the liver it is stored as glycogen. In the fat tissue it is stored as those love handles and beer belly you want to get rid of. When insulin is high, like after a high carbohydrate meal, it drives blood glucose into the liver to be converted into glycogen, which stops the use of fat as an energy source. When insulin is absent or low, glucose is not absorbed by most of the body cells and the body can then begin to use fat as an energy source. This is an oversimplification, but is nevertheless valid.

So how do we keep insulin from interfering with our weight loss 4 life? Have you heard of the glycemic index? The glycemic index ranks carbohydrates according to their effect on our blood sugar levels. High blood sugar levels trigger high insulin levels. The rating used to go from zero to one hundred but now I'm told it goes over 100. Sugar is on the high end of the scale as it is a simple molecule that triggers the immediate release of insulin. Carbohydrates with a lot of sugar raise the glycemic index to high levels creating that spike in insulin.

It is best to avoid high glycemic index carbohydrates when you're trying to burn body fat. If you want to learn more about the glycemic index go to glycemic index.com. Suffice it to say when your mom said eat your veggies, she was on to something. Vegetables are carbohydrates, but they are characteristically very, very low on the glycemic index scale whereas refined carbohydrates, like that bag of chips in your hand, are high on the glycemic index. Your mother was right, probably on more issues than I'm aware of, but specifically when it comes to veggies and the glycemic index. Most vegetables have a zero impact on blood sugar levels. I love salads because they keep my insulin levels stable, they hydrate me, and fill me up, thus curbing my appetite.

If you want to lose weight rapidly but not radically in the safe-and-sane approach, try replacing a lot of the high carbohydrate glycemic index foods that you eat with vegetables and lean meats. It's a simple approach to a lean body. Ask any bodybuilder; he or she will tell you that insulin turns off the fat burning switch and turns on the fat storage switch. For them that's bad enough, but it can also cause you to lose lean muscle mass. Those muscles are your engines that burn the fuel, so you don't want to lose lean muscle mass any more than they do!

When insulin brings down the blood sugar levels it often over corrects by causing low blood sugar. The body normally combats low blood sugar by releasing energy from stored fat, but the high level of insulin will not allow that to happen, so then the only source of energy is protein. When faced with this dilemma, your body will then break down muscle protein. Since it is a hybrid, it guarantees you won't starve, but it will cannibalize your muscles to keep you alive. It is a bad situation—gaining fat while at the same time losing lean muscle—and that's a lose-lose proposition. You can keep your insulin under control with a low glycemic diet, replacing the empty carbohydrates with vegetables and boosting the lean protein and good fats in your diet. Oh great! What are good fats? Don't worry, we'll get to that; relax, don't get your cortisol up.

Imagine that you're on the 91 freeway or if you live on the East Coast, imagine you're on the 95 freeway and suddenly a car cuts you off, slams on the brakes, and nearly causes an accident. What you're feeling right now is a hormone called adrenaline. Your body provides it for short-term stress. Now imagine that you're stuck on the freeway like the movie *Groundhog Day*, all day, every day, over and over again. What you begin to feel then is caused by the hormone cortisol, which is produced to help the body cope with mid-term stress. Cortisol is produced in the adrenal cortex and is released in response to stress to help prepare the body to react to potentially dangerous situations. It increases the level of sugar in the bloodstream and the brain's use of glucose while curbing nonessential bodily functions such as reproduction and growth and normal fat metabolism. Cortisol also suppresses the immune system and decreases the release of digestive secretions. Have you ever noticed that when you're stressed a glazed donut looks really good and promises to relieve that stress? Unless you're Bugs Bunny (and then a carrot might do it) we mortals crave sugary treats when cortisol is active in our bodies, which packs on the pounds. Your choice; avoid all stress or develop coping mechanisms for the stress that we all know is inevitable in this world.

Long-term stress, however, becomes an enemy rather than an ally. Stressful situations that last for an extended period of time, especially for those who have not discovered ways of coping with and letting go of their stress, will cause a continual release of cortisol, which will have many negative health effects such as anxiety, digestive troubles, heart disease, and weight gain. Good nutrition, good rest, and good exercise all limit cortisol's negative side effects. Any plan that is successful for life must include those three. Experts have also shown that music therapy—like smooth jazz—and massage therapy and meditation limit cortisol production as well.

Hopefully, you can begin to see that balance in all things is what will give you the results you desire. For example, good sleep not only allows you to wake up refreshed and less likely to move into the cortisol stress zone, it also releases a minor hormone known as leptin, which tells you that you have had enough to eat, and therefore, curbs your appetite.

Deep sleep and exercise also produce HGH or human growth hormone. HGH is involved in the conversion of body fat to muscle mass. Do I have your attention now? I thought so. It also plays an integral part in the growth of all tissues, in your energy level, tissue repair and body healing, cell replacement, bone strength, brain function, sexual function, and overall organ health and integrity, and the production of enzymes, hair, nails, and skin. Some have called it the fountain of youth. While it's not quite that simple, it is true that elevated HGH levels do make you feel young again. At twenty-years-old your body produces an average 500 micrograms per day of HDH; by the time you're eighty, you're down to about 25 mcg per day. This is why there's great interest in supplementation of HGH and/or diets that stimulate the natural production of HGH.

Why does your body produce less HGH as you get older? (If we had the answers to that, we could put a stop to aging right now!) Many believe it is much more complex than simply the levels of HGH and that it involves the length of the telomeres—the caps at the end of your DNA in every cell in your body. Evidence indicates that the telomeres seem to have a finite length and that the telomeres shorten each time you reproduce the cells to maintain your life. As you age they shorten and there is a greater chance of introducing errors into the reproduction of the cells. It's my theory that in the Garden of Eden, in the age of man's innocence on Earth, the "tree of life" bore fruit that provided telomerase releasing enzymes that kept us young indefinitely. But since it's not here anymore, what can we do? Well, perhaps we can find some other fruits or roots or vegetables that contain telomerase enzymes as well. In fact, that's been done. They are very rare and very expensive. It has also been demonstrated that spending a short time each day in an electric field of a certain frequency can also lengthen your telomeres over time.

But back to HGH. Some have resorted to injections of synthetic HGH to temporarily turn back the hands of time and convert body fat into muscle. It does work; however, there are also drawbacks and side effects. A better approach in dealing with HGH is, again, stress management; making sure you get the proper exercise at the proper levels and plenty of deep sleep. As we have already seen, these both promote the release of HGH. As we age we still produce HGH, but less and less is actually released into the body. Regular exercise and deep sleep in certain cycles prompt the release of your HGH. There are also some HGH stimulating formulas on the market that appear to be safe and moderately effective that cause your body to release your own natural HGH. Do you see the reoccurring theme? Regular exercise, especially resistance and interval training exercises, and sufficient deep sleep both release HGH.

Is it possible that all the ingredients for the mythical fountain of youth already exist within you? Is it possible that with good nutrition, good exercise, good rest, and a balanced lifestyle you can activate that fountain of youth within you?

The more we learn about the human organism the more we can see that nature has provided us with an incredible place to live; when we properly care for and keep everything in balance it functions as designed more often than not. As I mentioned earlier, one element of a balanced lifestyle is sufficient rest. During the rest cycle not only is HGH released but a minor hormone that suppresses appetite called leptin is also released. In a balanced internal environment leptin works together with another minor hormone called ghrelin, produced in your stomach when it's empty, to balance your appetite. Just like leptin, ghrelin goes into the blood, crosses the blood–brain barrier, and ends up in your hypothalamus.

Your brain perceives the difference in the mathematical equation between the balance of leptin versus ghrelin; if you want to lose weight, you want less ghrelin, so that you don't get those overpowering hunger pangs. Ghrelin levels are another reason to ensure you get the proper amount of rest for your body. It appears that with the proper amount of rest an adequate amount of leptin is released that counterbalances the ghrelin "hunger" hormone. As you can imagine, much research is still being done on these two hormones. It appears, though, that leptin is manufactured in the fat cells and released in the stomach and into the circulatory system where it travels to the hypothalamus and informs the brain that we have enough fat, so we can eat less. Some studies have indicated it may increase metabolism as well, but the one thing we know for certain: with inadequate rest, leptin is not released in effective amounts and the gremlin called ghrelin tips the scales in its own favor and creates hunger pangs.

Another little-known digestive hormone goes by the nickname of CCK; it's full name is Cholecystokinin. CCK is secreted by cells of the upper small intestine. It seems that it's secretion is stimulated by the introduction of HCl, amino acids, or fatty acids into the stomach or your duodenum. It may induce a feeling of fullness that is called SATIETY. It also appears to send a message to the hypothalamus indicating we are full and have no more need for food.

One more hormone we should take a look at is related to maintaining a healthy body weight, but also improves cognition and slows the aging process. Wow! It keeps you thin and it keeps you young, and last but not least, it keeps you smart—really! Irisin is a minor yet important hormone that is released after moderate endurance aerobic activity. The story is that one of the cell biologists who discovered the hormone irisin named it after Iris, the mythological Greek messenger goddess. The reason? Irisin seems to be a messenger hormone that appears to talk to various tissues in the body; it is released from muscle cells after endurance exercise and is somehow linked to triggering many of the health benefits of aerobic exercise. It appears that irisin is capable of reprogramming the body's fat cells to burn energy instead of storing it.

Experiments have shown that irisin levels increase as a result of a regular aerobic exercise, but not during short-term burst of anaerobic muscle activity. Irisin increases the metabolic rate; when irisin levels rise through aerobic exercise the hormone switches on genes that convert so-called white fat into so-called "good" brown fat. This is beneficial because "brown fat" continues to burn off more calories beyond the energy used (to do the actual aerobic exercise). In other words, it gives you a post exercise afterglow that continues to burn calories and helps you avoid obesity and conditions such as type II diabetes. This minor hormone, irisin, begins to look more like a major league player. Sounds to me like you better work in some aerobic exercises into your interval training as well, like tennis, cycling, speed walking, or jogging. I'm sure you'll think of something you can enjoy, because the aerobic exercise that stimulates the release of irisin improves cognitive function (your ability to think) and protects the brain against degeneration.

Do you remember the telomeres I recently mentioned, the protective end of the chromosomes that are made up of DNA and protein? Studies have shown that irisin has the ability to lengthen telomeres! Like the caps on the end of a shoelace, as they become shorter, their strength and structural integrity weakens, which causes the cells to age and die. It has been demonstrated that shorter telomeres are associated with a broad range of age-related diseases, including many forms of cancer, stroke, vascular dementia, cardiovascular disease, obesity, osteoporosis, and diabetes.

We have known for some time that exercise sharpens the mind and protects your overall health, but now it seems that we may have isolated one of the pathways and the hormone that activates that pathway—irisin. Are you beginning to see where I got the title for this book, *Weight Loss 4 Life*? Again we can see that a balanced lifestyle of proper rest, aerobic, interval, and resistance training exercise, and a good diet will not only give you a figure that you like to look at in the mirror, but will also make you smarter and allow you to live longer! Now that is weight loss 4 life!

Over the years I've been honored to meet and get to know some very famous bodybuilders; in fact, the best in the world. When it comes to building muscle and the physiology of fat loss, they are some of the wisest and most informed people on the planet. Any discussion of weight gain and weight loss, muscle gain and muscle loss, fat gain and fat loss cannot ignore the

600-pound gorilla in the room.

When it comes to hormones, the "big T" testosterone rules. Numerous studies have shown that simply by introducing "enough of the right steroid," testosterone levels will skyrocket, muscle growth will increase, and fat will disappear—all of this without exercise. Everyone knows that if you lift weights and train hard and you're on steroids, muscle growth will explode and fat will virtually disappear; clearly testosterone is very active in fat metabolism and muscle metabolism.

We also know that as well as friendly ones, steroids have unwanted side effects. Besides now being illegal in most jurisdictions, they are unsafe in most circumstances. In my opinion, they should be avoided unless medically indicated and recommended by your doctor. Some studies have shown that muscle growth doesn't change that dramatically even if your testosterone levels vary, as long as they are within the acceptable or normal physiological range for an adult male. On the other hand, researchers have found that fluctuations of testosterone within the physiological normal range had significant effects on body fat percentage. The higher the testosterone levels, the leaner the subjects were and conversely the lower the testosterone levels, the fatter they were. When researchers decreased certain subjects testosterone levels from the baseline average of 600 to around 300, they saw dramatic 36 percent increase in fat mass. So especially for men, although the exact mechanism isn't fully understood yet, researchers have shown that testosterone directly inhibits the creation of fat cells and low testosterone is a contributing factor to obesity.

The take-away is: doing things to naturally increase your testosterone levels can help you get and stay lean. However, if you want to become Mr. Olympia you first need to find a jurisdiction that allows you to legally get medical help and hormones that boost your testosterone 20 - 30 percent above the normal physiological range. Then in the presence of extreme protein diets and extreme workouts, you will pack on muscle and perhaps be well on your way to a Mr. or Ms. Olympia title.

But that's not what we're after, right? We are after weight loss 4 life, so there's no need to move to another country and become the Incredible Hulk to achieve fat loss with testosterone boosting supplements. There are numerous over-the-counter legal testosterone boosting supplements available. Many of them have liver and kidney detoxifying factors, estrogen control factors, and nitric oxide boosters as well as the natural herbs that boost testosterone. None of these will take you outside the normal range and turn you into Mr. Olympia. But they will increase your testosterone within the normal physiological range, which will decrease your fat and perhaps decrease your recovery time if you're also a weightlifting athlete.

As with any hormone, it is wise to be under a doctor's care and direction when you set out to modify its concentration in your system. Remember, endocrinology is like a three- or four-dimensional chess game; every move you make affects numerous other hormones in your system. The wisest thing one can do is seek to normalize all the values of all the different hormones in your body and keep them normal. This is most often accomplished—yes, you guessed it—with proper rest, proper nutrition, proper exercise, and sometimes proper supplementation, but always balance in all things.

Here are a few safe and sane and healthy ways to boost your testosterone naturally.

Number one: eat the right vegetables

Remember that we said vegetables are good carbohydrates? Cruciferous vegetables such as bok choy, broccoli, Brussels sprouts, cabbage, cauliflower, kale, etc., can reduce estrogen by 50 percent, which in turn helps maintain optimum levels of testosterone. Work at least one to two servings of these veggies into your daily meal plan

Number two: eat more meat (or protein)

Now I'm a vegetarian so I don't eat meat, but I do increase my protein intake from quality sources, including protein supplements.

Number three: eat healthy fats

I told you we would come back to those healthy fats. They are the densest energy source available to your body. Each gram of fat contains over twice the calories of a gram of carbohydrate or protein. Healthy fats such as those found in dairy, olive oil, avocados, flaxseeds, and many nuts are actually an important component to overall health. So-called healthy fats help your body absorb the other nutrients that you give it, and nourish the nervous system as well as help maintain cell structures, regulate hormone levels, and more.

One category of fats you want to avoid, though, are the trans fats. Trans fats are the modified form of the saturated fat that's been engineered to give foods longer shelf life and certain flavors. Many cheap processed and packaged foods are full of trans fats; check the labels and AVOID them!

Number four: chill out

If your testosterone levels are suppressed and other hormone levels are inflated, such as cortisol, you need to take a break, slow down, breathe deeply, and process your stress so that you can let go of it. I've shared with you that exercise is my favorite way of meditating, followed closely by Centerpoint's Holosync® technology. I'm certain you will find many techniques that will work for you.

Number five: get enough sleep

If you're not getting enough sleep you will suppress your testosterone levels and will elevate your cortisol levels. Since I've introduced you to leptin, you already know one of the reasons you need seven to nine hours sleep per night. This is an important time for your entire body, including your endocrine system, to recover, heal, and normalize itself.

Number six: have sex

It is not a myth that for both male and females having sex at least once a week keeps testosterone levels higher. It's science and in this case, more is better.

Number seven: take supplements

- Make sure you're getting from 1000 to 1500 mg of a good source of vitamin C per day. Also, many studies have shown that 250 to 500 mg of ginseng daily is especially helpful for women. Make sure your supplement contains zinc, magnesium, and vitamin B6 as well as other vitamins and minerals from a natural source. I recommend and take:

- 60 essential minerals

- 16 essential vitamins

- 12 essential amino acids

- 3 essential fatty acids

We will talk a bit more about an "ideal" diet and supplementation programs in Chapter 6. Recognize the fact that we are all individuals and as such, there is no cookie cutter answer, but there are guiding principles that will be of benefit to everyone. It is my intent to equip you with the information and tools so that you can customize your individual stylized plan of... weight loss 4 life. For long life and health!

Chapter 3: What About a Detox as a Jump Start?

Several years ago I had the privilege of traveling to a beautiful resort in Fiji. This wasn't just any resort; it was Namale, an exclusive resort owned by Tony Robbins. Yes, *that* Tony Robbins. I had the honor of meeting him there and staying in the Bourae (cabin/condo) that's next to his house at the resort. In different buildings around the resort you see pictures and comments from celebrities who have come to visit and have enjoyed Tony's hospitality.

But I wasn't one of those celebrities. I was there with his life mastery class. My son and I signed up for his Mastery University. We participated in one of his famous "fire walks," which is really quite a dramatic event—walking across hot coals glowing at over 1000°—not feeling a thing and sustaining no damage really shows you our internal potential. We really can do just about anything we put our minds to... but we will come to that in Chapter 7.

I don't know what I expected but it certainly wasn't what was waiting for us. Yes, we had an out-of-the-box climb up a huge telephone pole on top of a hill overlooking the ocean. We, well most of us, climbed all the way to the top, then negotiated a way to climb onto and stand on the top of the eight- to ten-inch diameter end of the pole as it swayed back and forth seemingly in the stratosphere. Then we jumped off from a height that would kill us if our safety equipment did not work. It was an exercise to take us outside our comfort zone and it worked!

I did expect something like that, but I didn't expect what came next. After getting to know his staff, I found out they call it the "Last Supper" and while it isn't followed by a crucifixion, the next day begins some serious self-sacrifice as we are introduced to Tony's detox plan.

I had never really thought that I needed any of the many cleanses or detox plans that are bantered about in public forums. I was a lifelong vegetarian, an athlete, and I took good care of myself. I didn't take any prescription medications, I didn't eat weird exotic unclean meats from Timbuktu with a high potential for tapeworms and who knows what else in them. It just seemed like a waste of time to me. It didn't take me long to see that Tony believed that everyone could benefit from his detox and cleanse program. The last supper consisted of a veritable banquet of beautiful multicolored vegetables of every kind. We were told we could have as much as we wanted. It was fresh and inviting with guacamole to dip the veggies in.

Then came the catch. We were told that the next day we would start a detox program consisting largely of wheatgrass juice and something called Udo's oil, occasionally some broth to balance our electrolytes, hot-spa treatments and massages, (okay, it was beginning to sound better), and then something called colonics. Someone asked what that was.

The instructor described the procedure and I said, "You put what, where"?

He responded with a laugh. "That is exactly what Tony said the first time he was introduced to it and now he swears by its health benefits."

I thought to myself, really? Well, I had just seen him that morning and he looked fine, actually pretty healthy and big and strong to me. Apparently it didn't kill him; I guess I could survive it.

Bright and early the next morning we met in the lecture hall, which had a spectacular view of the tropical sea laying at the bottom of the cliff below. We had a few minutes to get to know each other and exchange pleasantries with leaders from all over the world who had gathered there for that week. Then they brought us our breakfasts: two-ounce shots of wheatgrass. I had mine and thought it wasn't too bad, though it would have been better with some scrambled eggs and salsa on the side.

For the next couple hours we sat through one expert after another telling us the benefits of live foods. Having studied history I was acutely aware of the fact that Fiji used to be home to cannibals. The people I met were terrific, friendly, wonderful people, but I began to wonder what they meant by 'live' food?! Well, it turns out that wheatgrass is considered a live food. It is grown and cultivated and then squeezed and turned into juice and then consumed immediately thereafter. When consumed in this manner it contains a litany of healthful ingredients that some people say can cure any disease and if you don't have one, it can prevent them. I was sure glad that it is so good for us because it certainly was not going to win any taste tests.

After a couple more hours of lectures we had lunch, which consisted of more shots of wheatgrass and something called Udo's oil that we had just learned was a perfect blend of omega three, six, and nine oils. It turns out that every cell, tissue, gland, and organ in our body is dependent upon the presence of essential fatty acids. They are the main structural components of cell membranes and are necessary for cell growth and division. I remembered from my research for another book that cell membranes were actually the cells' brains (unlike what we had been taught in biology that it was in the nucleus), so I listened carefully. I learned that Udo's oil was formulated by Udo Erasmus, PhD, an internationally acclaimed authority on the subject of essential fatty acids and author of a great book called *Fats That Heal, Fats That Kill*. I was impressed! Dr. Erasmus developed this blend to detoxify himself after he was exposed to some potentially lethal contaminants. About a year later I met Dr. Erasmus in Nassau, Bahamas, and thanked him for sharing his discovery with the world. I didn't thank him for the taste so much or the fine bouquet of the oil, but what it lacked in flavor it made up for in potency. For those who can't get past the taste, it now comes in softgels. I recommend them.

Before I knew it the afternoon of lectures had

passed and we were enjoying our abbreviated gourmet supper of wheatgrass and Udo's oil. Later that night, I drifted off to sleep in my very comfortable bed with the sound of tropical seas rolling in upon the shore, and thought, "Well, I made it through day one and they haven't kicked me off the island yet."

Not only did Tony's program include live foods, detoxification, good fats, education, exercise, meditation, and relaxation in the spa— including massages, there were those dreaded colonics as well. It turned out that they weren't so bad after all. The beautiful island days came and went and before we realized it many of us had become more than friends. In fact, we had become family, a family that came from all over the world.

As we listened to lectures on our last day, many of us were jumping up and down (on the rebounders) with excitement that the fast was nearly over. Actually, jumping was part of the program. There were enough rebounders— small trampolines—that we each had our own that we could use any time we wanted to wake ourselves up. And yes, you guessed it, there are a lot of health benefits to rebounding that I will share with you in Chapter 4.

The instructor asked if we had noticed any positive results from our six days on the island. I guess he didn't want to hear about the nights our stomachs growled, or maybe he had already heard that. Seriously, we had all done quite well and as the testimonies started to roll in, we found that not only had we survived the six day live food detox cleanse and fast, many of us were feeling energized and more alive and yes, even though we had not intended to, many of us had lost weight. I lost fourteen pounds and I wasn't even aware of it until they made the scales available to us. I must say that when I got home and looked at the pictures of me playing volleyball without a shirt on our final day, I could tell. I looked pretty good, like high school except with more muscle. (I like to lift weights.) Thank you, Tony!

Just like Tony intended, my week on the island was a paradigm shifting event. I now believe there is a time and a place for a well-balanced cleanse or detox and live foods in my life. I still look for a place where I can get at least a two-ounce shot of wheatgrass every day, and now that I am rehabbing from an injury—eight ounces! A couple of years after returning from my experience in Fiji I addressed another Tony Robbins event; this time in Palm Springs. I shared with them the lasting positive results that I had from my week in Fiji. As I looked at the couple of thousand faces—many of them staring back at me blankly—I said that I knew how they felt as they were right in the middle of that week-long experience and I had a little bit of empathy. I encouraged them not to give up, that it would be worth it, and that even now— several years later—wherever I went I still got my two-ounce shot of wheatgrass. In fact, even at Disneyland there is a Jamba Juice (in between California Adventure and the parking lot) and they have fresh wheatgrass juice. I assured them that there was no reason and no excuse not to keep going. I also shared with them a couple of humorous stories that occurred in Fiji and as I spoke I began to notice life come back into their faces—or maybe it was just my face in the mirror—because that night I overcame my fear of public speaking. Again, thank you, Tony!

If you have never done a detox or cleanse in your life, it may be a great way to start your journey back to ideal health. If you are like me and think that live food might mean you're on the menu, let me reassure you: you're not. But I recommend that you add wheatgrass to your diet daily; after all, look what it does for cows and those big Brahma bulls. No weakness there! Good news: you won't have to chew it like they do. Jamba juice or your local vitamin or health food store will juice it right there for you and you can drink it in a couple seconds or less. It is actually kind of sweet! Let me take a few moments and share with you the incredible benefits of wheatgrass juice.

Studies have shown that wheatgrass can be an effective healer, because it contains virtually all the minerals known to man and vitamins A, B complex, C, E, and K. It is extremely rich in protein and contains 17 amino acids that can be used to build other proteins as the body needs them. Wheatgrass juice can contain up to 70 percent chlorophyll. The chlorophyll molecule closely resembles that of the hemin molecule, the pigment that combines with protein to form hemoglobin in human blood. The major difference between the chlorophyll molecule and the hemoglobin molecule is that the chlorophyll molecule contains magnesium as its central atom, and the hemin molecule contains iron. The molecular structure of these two substances are almost identical in all other respects.

Chlorophyll contains enzymes and super oxidase dismutase, a copper containing protein found in mature red blood cells. This enzyme decomposes superoxide radicals in the body into a more manageable form, therefore helping to slow down the aging process. Chlorophyll is virtually the first product of light, therefore contains more light energy or photons than any other food element; at least that's what scientists tell us. Science has also shown that chlorophyll arrests the growth and development of unfriendly bacteria. In other words, chlorophyll is antibacterial and can be used inside and outside the body as a natural healer.

In the early years of the atomic energy program the United States Army exposed guinea pigs to lethal doses of radiation. Guinea pigs fed the chlorophyll rich vegetables had half the mortality rate as those fed non-chlorophyll diets. It would appear that it is a strong antioxidant as well. It has also been shown that chlorophyll neutralizes toxins in the body, helps purify the liver, improves blood sugar imbalances, and washes away residual drug deposits from the body.

Wheatgrass contains a full spectrum of vitamins and minerals and it has been reported that farmers in the know put their sterile cows and bulls on wheatgrass to restore their fertility.

Apparently the high magnesium content in the chlorophyll builds enzymes that restore the sex hormones. Wheatgrass is literally the stuff from which legends are made, the proverbial magic bullet. It is considered a nutritionally complete food for animals and humans alike. Some of the other benefits of consuming wheatgrass juice are an increase in the red blood cell count, it cleanses the blood and organs and the gastrointestinal track, it stimulates metabolism, and it also stimulates your thyroid gland! It's also reported to reduce the over acidity in your blood to relieve peptic ulcers, ulcerative colitis, and constipation. It contains the enzyme SOD, an anti-inflammatory compound, which might be one reason the guinea pigs exposed to radiation did better with wheatgrass juice afterwards. While I'm not convinced that wheatgrass is my favorite food choice, there is no doubt in my mind that it can play a significant role in optimal nutrition.

Wheatgrass juice is not alone. You can gain a lot from juicing your vegetables as well. By juicing you allow yourself the ability to consume a larger variety of vegetables and more vegetables per day. This is important because most people don't eat enough vegetables. Juicing and drinking your vegetables first thing in the morning can give you a natural energy boost without resorting to stimulants like coffee. Since juice is already in an easily digestible form, it can help revitalize your energy levels within as little as twenty minutes. Suffice it to say that juicing wheatgrass and other vegetables, beans, nuts, seeds, and grains can be a great benefit to your health. They are an important support for cell regeneration and a powerful source of antioxidants, minerals, vitamins, and enzymes that protects the body against free radical damage, and they also have an alkalizing effect on your body, which has a protective effect against diseases, including cancer. We will talk more about this in Chapter 6.

If you thought this was a brand new scientific revelation, let me remind you that over 2000 years ago Hippocrates, the father of modern medicine, said, "Let food be thy medicine and medicine be thy food." He also said, "If we could give every individual the right amount of nourishment and exercise, not too little and not too much, we would have found the safest way to health." One might legitimately ask if the statement of a physician nearly 2500 years ago holds any credibility in this age of scientific enlightenment. That's a good question.

While it is true that we've made incredible scientific advancements in just the last 60 years, more than the last thousands put together, is it not possible that we have lost something as well? When beautiful palaces are built on a strong foundation they will endure time and the elements. Same is true with our health. Hippocrates laid a strong foundation that we in medicine seem to have forgotten. As with a beautiful palace that has added central air and indoor plumbing and even Wi-Fi, we have updated and supposedly upgraded our bodies (palaces) with modern diets, modern pharmaceuticals, and a modern pace of life that has caused us to largely forget our foundations.

But what about our foundation? We once understood that food is a medicine and as such bad food is bad medicine and it will make us sick. Good food is good medicine and it can make us well if we are sick, perhaps even reversing and curing some diseases, and prevent us from catching others. Unfortunately, today some of our scientists have become so myopic focusing on their new discoveries that they regard the simple formula of taking away bad food and putting in good food as magic, but they won't hesitate to offer you a drug to cure your skin rash that will give you half a dozen side effects and two or three other diseases in the process.

Please don't misunderstand me. We have rightfully built a place for pharmacology in the ivory towers of our modern medicine, but no tower can stand without its foundation and as far back as Hippocrates we knew that foundation was good nutrition. Let your food be your medicine and let your medicine be your food.

My father was a chemist who held numerous patents. Some of those patents saved many, many lives. But with the advent of the age of medicinal chemicals has come the increase in toxic chemicals as well. Many authorities believe that life in the 21st century is very toxic and that this is one of the reasons for the epidemic of obesity in the world today. They claim that our diets have become toxic with volumes of empty calories that do not provide the nutrition our bodies need, but do contain chemicals and additives that cause us to want more and more and more calories. As evidence, you have all seen the commercial for a potato chip brand not so long ago that said, "Bet you can't eat just one." I tried; they won that bet. A good case can be made for periodically evaluating our diets for nutritional content and purity, and then, detox our bodies periodically. They insist that in doing so we remove the toxic roadblocks to absorbing good nutrition, thereby performing much-needed maintenance on our foundation.

When my computer gets too many windows open and is overloaded with empty programs and is too congested with cookies—and I'm referring to computer cookies—it is beneficial to restart it to improve its performance. Perhaps the same is true of our internal computers. I think a case can be made for periodic safe and sane detox diets that take us back to natural foods, where our foods truly can be our medicines, and our medicines our foods.

At the beginning of the chapter I shared with you my experience with Tony Robbins and his recommended detoxing cleanse at his Fiji resort and briefly described his detox regimen. There are elements of his plan that I still do daily. In Chapter 6, I'll share some of those with you, as well as some supplements that work for me. I will also include input from Dr. Neumann, my wife and physician, who has successfully helped many patients lose weight and detox their bodies, and from my sons

Adam, Jonathan, and Craig Luckey, all active not only in the fitness industry but in a holistic approach to wellness.

You remember that in my visit to Tony Robbins' resort in Fiji, I found out that in addition to being a proponent of live foods and wheatgrass and Udo's oil, Tony also believed in colonics for detoxifying the body. Some people believe that colonics or colon hydrotherapy are only necessary for those who have been exposed to known toxicities, very poor diets, or have digestive symptoms.

Proponents of colon hydrotherapy say it is a safe and highly effective method to cleanse the large intestines of accumulated waste and rancid toxins. I recommend a Libby system as Tony did. During a colonic, filtered water is introduced into the colon, softening and loosening waste to be evacuated through peristalsis (smooth muscle contractions). It is said that colon hydrotherapy permits other organs of elimination such as the skin, lungs, liver, and kidneys to function more effectively, which provides detoxification of the cells throughout the body to improve absorption and assimilation of nutrients throughout the body. Again, the proponents of colon hydrotherapy say that most people are carrying around more than five undigested meals in their digestive systems! Among others things, this can cause their abdomens to distend with discomfort. This waste material is rancid and can be reabsorbed by the intestines causing the onset of other health conditions over time. It is claimed that colonics help relieve common conditions of constipation, bloating, heartburn, acid reflex, and reduce stress as well.

No one would argue that a healthy colon will help support and improve your overall health; the questions come when we begin to determine what it is we have to do to maintain a healthy colon. Many people say that whenever they feel a cold or flu coming on that's the first thing they turn to, to avoid the disease process.

So how does all this fit into weight loss? Well, clearly, if you're carrying around part of some of the meals that you've eaten long ago, that dead weight will tip the scales and not in your favor. If you can eliminate that waste material you will not only lose weight, but you will improve the function of your digestive system and if you maintain a regular elimination of that waste material you won't regain that weight, either. If you decide this might be beneficial weight- or health-wise to you, I suggest you search online for a Libby equipped colon hydrotherapy salon in your area.

I believe that any time your body is working at its optimum, your mind-body-spirit matrix works more efficiently, which includes not carrying excess weight. I personally prefer the Aqua Chi; it's a little more relaxing and a lot less invasive and that works for me. If you don't need a colonic, it's a less invasive way to energize and detoxify your body. The Aqua Chi is the world's leader in ionic foot spa technology. The negative ions created and absorbed during an Aqua chi foot spa session are similar to those found in hot springs and other naturally charged water sources that have been shown to be beneficial to the body. I love it and wouldn't be without one. If you're interested, you can find more information online; I recommend that you look for the original Aqua Chi system.

Chapter 4: You Got to Move it, Move it, if Ya Want to Lose it, Lose it!

"I like to Move it - Move it." If you have children, then you already know that this is the theme of a song showcased by DreamWorks in the Madagascar series of animated films. No matter what branch of the animal kingdom you belong to, you got to move it -move it! So, why not make it a dance and have fun with it like the characters in the movie do?

It is ironic that as I wrote this chapter of the book I was incapacitated. My right hip was diagnosed as having arthritis and was causing unbearable pain, affecting every aspect of my life. To add insult to injury, I had a broken finger and ruptured tendon and a splint on my ring finger of my right hand! Ironically, I injured it demonstrating how not to injure your fingers while preforming a martial arts move that I have done for 40 years. This time I showed them how *not* to do it. I do not recommend that teaching technique.

It does, however, provide for another teaching moment. Variety. Fill your life with variety. Treat yourself to a variety of healthy foods, and yes, cultivate a wide variety of activities and sports that will provide you with the exercise you need—sometimes without even realizing it. My dad used to say he loved playing tennis because in his love for the game he didn't even realize he was exercising. I share his love for tennis, but clearly these crutches and the splint on my racket hand really hindered my movement around the court. Consider that reason number one to cultivate different forms of exercise. In my case, after taking a break from writing, I headed to the gym and lifted weights. The truth is, if you live long enough you're going to experience some injuries in your life that will interfere with your favorite forms of exercise. I am glad that I had a plan B, C, D, and E in store for just a time like this.

It's so easy for us humans to become stalled by legitimate detours in our lives and allow them to become excuses for inactivity and non-movement. Maybe you just had a baby and you can't go play tennis, either. Well, the other day I was down by the beach and saw a new mother jogging with her baby in the stroller. By the expression on her face she was loving it… the fresh air, the salt breeze… just getting out and being able to move again put a smile on her face. Detours are not stop signs. They simply require that we take a different course than the one we intended to pursue. Into every life detours will come, and for that reason I suggest you prepare ahead of time so that your detours do not become stop signs. Take a lesson from the GPS in your car or your smart phone; have a few alternative routes ready when life throws those detours at you. When an injury comes don't sit down and cry in your protein drink; reach for plan B or C or even D so that you can safely keep moving - moving because you got to move it - move it. Listen as your internal GPS says, "Recalculating course" and follow it to your desired destination: weight loss 4 life.

I'm sure you recall from previous chapters that there is another good reason to embrace a variety of different exercises in your lifestyle. You recall that aerobic exercise releases a hormone called irisin, right? Do you remember all the good things it does? Quick refresher: irisin rejuvenates your telomeres and keeps you young. It also enhances your cognition and mental abilities, and of course, helps keep you thin and fit for life. Boy, could I use a long set of tennis right now! However, those crutches are still sitting right next to me and if I turn even a little bit to look at them my right hip will remind me why we're not playing tennis today.

But I have some good news. If you want to move your strength training to a level of endurance training, thereby gaining aerobic benefits, you can do that. Just lighten up your weights and cut down your rest time between sets and you will begin to add the benefits of aerobic training to your strength training. So now I'm combining the benefits of both forms of exercise and making the best out of my detour. You may recall that strength training (lifting weights for me) will facilitate the release of growth hormone, build my muscles, which are the engines that burn the calories, release endorphins that make me feel better even if my situation hasn't changed for the better yet, and strengthen my bones and ligaments and tendons, preventing osteoporosis from inactivity. Today I am going to decrease my weights, so that I can decrease my time between sets, so that I can push my resistance strength training into the endurance and aerobic exercise realm as well. I'm expecting my body will produce irisin for me now as well.

Detours will come, but you just have to keep moving and not let those detours steal your joy. When detours arise it is normal to experience disappointment and easy to allow that disappointment to turn into depression. It turns out, though, that exercise is one of your best weapons against depression. Detours come with plenty of stress and anxiety and if you're already overweight with resulting low self-esteem it's easy for depression to set in. The first thing you have to do is to exercise your intellectual and emotional intelligence and simply tell yourself you're not going to allow that to happen to you. Research has shown that moderate exercise is one of the quickest and best ways to avoid depression. For instance, when a person exercises, levels of both circulating serotonin and endorphins are increased rapidly. These hormones help fight off depression, and the really good news is that their levels stay elevated for several days after exercise is discontinued. Clearly, if you want to feel better and avoid depression, moderate exercise is the best prescription. Even if you miss a day or two you may not have a major letdown if you get right back at it.

Another good reason not to let the detours of life stop you from exercising is that when you exercise you sleep better—unless you exercise right before you try to go to sleep; not recommended. The ideal time to exercise is probably four to eight hours before you sleep. Remember we learned in a previous chapter how important it is to get good sleep. During deep sleep cycles hormones such as HGH are released that balance our systems and prevent obesity.

In addition to enhancing deep sleep and counteracting depression, exercise improves brain function and reduces the risk of developing dementia. Part of that is due to the increased blood and oxygen flow to the brain; increased growth factors that are released promote synaptic plasticity and create new nerve cells, which we know helps with cognition through the release of chemicals such as dopamine, glutamate, norepinephrine, serotonin, and other endorphins and hormones. Unless you're training for a marathon, evidence indicates that moderate exercise has a beneficial effect on the human immune system as well. In this case too much of a good thing might not be so good and extreme athletes can actually lower their immunity by not allowing enough time for the body to rebuild after the stresses of exercise. Again the key is balance; consistent moderate exercise offers all the benefits.

The beneficial effects of moderate exercise on the cardiovascular system are well documented. So is the direct relationship between physical inactivity and cardiovascular mortality. If you're sedentary and physically inactive there is great potential to reduce your mortality due to cardiovascular disease by becoming moderately active on a regular basis; in other words, you got to move it - move it! Both aerobic and anaerobic or resistance exercise work to increase the mechanical efficiency of the heart by increasing cardiac volume and myocardial thickness; they give you a stronger heart.

Of course you know by now that physical exercise is important for maintaining physical and emotional fitness and wellness and can contribute to positively maintaining a healthy weight and building and maintaining healthy bone density, muscle strength, and joint mobility. Now we know that it promotes physiological and psychological well-being and enhances the immune system. But here's another nice benefit of exercise; it also reduces the level of cortisol. Remember, cortisol is a stress hormone that builds fat in the abdominal region, making weight loss difficult. Cortisol causes many other health problems, both physical and emotional. It's a fact that frequent and regular exercise has been shown to help prevent and treat serious life-threatening chronic conditions such as high blood pressure, obesity, heart disease, type II diabetes, insomnia, and of course the other "d" that follows the detours so often—depression.

So now you know, don't stop and give up when the injuries and detours of life present themselves; instead, prepare now intellectually emotionally and physically for alternatives when the detour signs appear. Program your GPS with a cornucopia of fun, exciting, and healthful ways to exercise so that even when the injuries come you do not have to give up the benefits that regular exercise gives you free of charge.

Let's look at some options and what they do for you:

Let's start with tennis. You may not realize it, but a good hour of tennis will burn about 600 calories and is going to increase your aerobic capacity, lower your resting heart rate and blood pressure, improve metabolic function, increase bone density, lower your body fat, improve muscle tone and strength and flexibility, and increase your reaction times. In a good set of tennis there are a lot of stops and starts and sprints, standing, and walking, which really makes it a good interval training sport.

The interval training aspect pushes it higher on my list of favorites—above jogging and cycling or even an indoor cycling class—and like my dad said, it'll be the fastest hour of your day. Bjorn Borg once said tennis is a match of "1000 little sprints." The quick anaerobic movements that the sport demands burns fat, increases your heart rate, and promotes higher energy levels, and yes, you're right… I miss it.

Cycling, either riding a bicycle outside—which has the additional benefits of fresh air—or a lifecycle in a gym or at home is another good option. Cycling can increase your cardiovascular fitness by 3 to 7 percent. Cycling uses the largest muscle groups, the legs. Raising your heart rate to benefit stamina and fitness is a good way to lose some unwanted pounds and it burns about 300 calories per hour at a steady pace. If you want to work it like the Tour de France you can boost that number up considerably. It is not jarring or hard on the joints and is something you can do all your life, barring injuries. The list of benefits is very close to that of tennis and includes cardiovascular fitness, increased muscle strength and flexibility, improved joint mobility, and decreased stress levels, along with improved posture and coordination—or decreased posture, depending on your bike set up—strengthened bones and decreased body fat levels.

Another great racket sport I enjoy is racquetball. If tennis, as Bjorn Borg says, is a match of 1000 "little sprints," then racquetball is a game of 2000 even smaller sprints. Like tennis, racquetball improves your coordination and your balance, strengthens your heart, maintains bone density, and is a great total body workout. Depending on your weight and the level of intensity with which you play, you can expect to burn 600 to 800 calories per hour playing racquetball.

Remember the mom I saw pushing a stroller ahead of her as she jogged along the beach? I'm sure it was a great mental health break for her. Let's take a look at the other health benefits that she's gaining as she jogs. I consider running one of the best types of exercise. I guess that goes back quite a ways; I can remember my mom saying she thinks I was born running! Clearly, with a hip injury I'm not running right now and I do miss it.

My favorite form of running are short sprints followed by short recovery periods. I consider 10s or 15s, as we used to call them, or interval sprints as one of the best fat burning and overall conditioning exercises out there, and it's simple; you just sprint ten yards, stop, touch the ground and sprint back the other way ten yards, stop, touch the ground and sprint back in the other direction; fifteen yards, etc., etc. One advantage is you don't need any athletic gear, just an open field where you can measure off the distance you want to sprint and that's it. I recommend them If you're in pretty good shape. If you have a high school track available to you, you can also run "sprint and walks." They are just as they sound: sprints followed by walks, followed by sprints, followed by walks. Often we ran the turns and walked the straightaway or vice versa; you can do that at your own pace.

Speaking of at our own pace, let's get back to jogging.

To me, jogging was always a warm-up before the workout, but right now with my injured hip, I would be happy to be able to go jogging for a half hour at any pace. It has been shown that regular jogging not only improves cardiovascular fitness but indeed has mental health benefits such as helping to manage depression and anxiety. Regular running and jogging is a good way to improve your overall health and fitness and help you lose weight; you don't need to become a marathon runner to benefit greatly from running or jogging. I would recommend getting good quality running shoes. You want to do everything you can to protect your knees and hips and ankles, etc.

If you find yourself out of breath, don't stop altogether; keep walking. As long as you're moving, you're burning calories and still receiving the many benefits of exercise. Depending on your weight, jogging will burn around 600 calories per hour. Walking will still burn around 300 calories per hour. If the scenery is getting boring for you, or you simply don't have a safe place to run or jog or walk, another great alternative is an aerobics class at a local gym. Research shows that you can burn from 400 to 500 calories per hour in a low impact cardio or aerobics class at your local gym. One benefit of an aerobics class is that you can build friendships and camaraderie with others pursuing common goals, perhaps even build positive peer pressure and accountability that will help keep your exercise consistent. There is usually some good music to keep you moving and the time goes faster than if you spend an hour jogging or walking, though some people prefer the peace and quiet of a walk in nature or a jog where they can relax into a hypnotic rhythm and pace and lose track of time as well. The point is to find something that you enjoy and do it consistently. Authentic weight loss 4 life can be fun. There's no reason for it to become boring, because there are so many options.

Speaking of not being bored, have you ever tried a boot camp? No, I'm not recruiting for the Marine Corps, though I respect them greatly. The boot camp experience is never boring and it often incorporates resistance training as well as aerobic training and stretching, pretty much a buffet of all the different varieties of exercise in one place at one time. As we saw earlier, interval training like that is one of the quickest ways to burn fat. Just don't let the name boot camp intimidate you. You're not going to have an overbearing staff sergeant with bad breath yelling in your face or kicking your backside if you're not moving fast enough. Just listen to your body and go at your own pace. Studies show that you will burn 600 calories in 45 minutes! It seems that you will burn more calories in less time and you won't be bored.

Let me encourage you to go online to the Mayo Clinic or Livestrong or just google, "How many calories will I burn in an hour of____"; then fill in the blank with the exercise you're interested in. There are many sites that offer more precise calorie burn rates where you can individualize your results with your weight, your age, etc. Let me also encourage you not to become overly focused on the math. Whatever you do—enjoy it—have fun and don't let anything steal your joy!

It is not my purpose to turn you into a miserly calorie counting nag, but rather an educated and enlightened individual who enjoys the dance of life! When we watch great athletes like Usain Bolt run the hundred or 200 meter or Michael Jordan in his prime playing basketball it all looks so incredibly easy. I guarantee you that even with their talent, they didn't start at the top; when their game sputtered they went back to the basics. That's what I'm teaching you here—the basics. Learn them, but don't focus on them; rather, focus on the joy of movement and the freedom of exercise. If you're not getting the results you want, then go back and review your basics by checking the amount and quality of your fuel sources and diet and balance that with more or less exercise as needed. Just keep it fun; it's not brain surgery.

As for fun, I'm about to take a break and go

jump on a trampoline. I'll tell you all the great benefits of it when I get back.

When my daughter was young we bought her a full-size trampoline and set it up in the back yard. When she was a little older she became a flyer on a world champion competitive cheer team. I must admit I felt a lot more relaxed when I watched her twenty feet in the air over a trampoline than I did over the outstretched arms of two other girls promising to catch her on the way down. But it never seemed to bother her. She learned to fly when she was just a little girl, and honestly, I had a lot of fun with it, too, as did her big brothers who were bodybuilding, record-breaking, scholarship making, football players.

It wasn't until I spent that week in Fiji at Tony Robbins' resort that I found out how good all that play on the trampoline was for us. As I mentioned earlier, Tony had designed his beautiful lecture room overlooking the azure tropical seas below with mini trampolines so that, at any time—even during lectures—if we felt fatigued or just wanted to speed up our heart rate, we were encouraged to jump on the trampolines. Tony and his instructors knew that it was better to have somebody wide awake jumping on a trampoline listening to them than somebody sitting in a chair nodding off.

Jumping on a mini-trampoline, or rebounding, may not be your idea of a strenuous aerobic exercise and it may not have occurred to you that it has significant health benefits, but in fact both are true. In fact, this benign, safe form of gentle-no impact exercise actually burns more calories than jogging! It can be adjusted to your fitness level, it's easy on your joints and back, and it can be done in your home at your convenience. I have a mini trampoline in the back yard; it's about three feet in diameter, just like the ones Tony has in his resort in Fiji.

One of the first things I do in the morning is make my way out into the fresh air and onto the mini trampoline, and like the song says, move it-move it. Studies have shown that rebounding reduces back and joint pain, alleviates arthritic symptoms, such as pain and inflammation, and boosts energy levels. Rebounding is sufficiently gentle so that nearly everyone can participate. Before I took a break, my hip was beginning to hurt even as I simply sat here and wrote about fitness. But now there is a warm glowing feeling where that pain once was. Rebounding is a unique exercise in that you achieve a weightless state at the top of each jump, then land with twice the force of gravity on each bounce. This twice-gravity bounce affects every muscle and cell of the body in a positive manner.

One of rebounding's special benefits is its ability to stimulate the flow of the lymphatic system. Your lymph system depends on physical motion and activity to circulate fluids. The rebounding motion is the perfect exercise for your lymph system. Stagnant or inadequate lymph flow is associated with the onset of many symptoms and underlying illnesses including bursitis in the shoulders, general joint stiffness, and soft-tissue spasms. It is vital that the lymph fluids continue to flow in order to eliminate waste from the body; without a pump like the heart, that flow is dependent on muscle contractions and body movements and gravity.

The list of positive benefits resulting from rebounding is long and legendary and I'll let you explore it at your leisure. The entire cosmos is in motion. From the smallest subatomic particles right inside your body to the largest stars of the universe, millions of light years away, a quantum dance is in progress. Why not get up off the couch, listen for the music, and join in the party?

You got to move it - move it!

Chapter 5: What's Eating You?

Most books written for and about weight loss and diet focus on just that: your diet. Of course what you are eating, the volume, the timing, and the types of food are of great importance, but sometimes it is really about what's eating you! Do you remember the last time you received some deeply profound emotionally disturbing news? Perhaps you checked your retirement portfolio at lunch and the stock market had just crashed. Was that terrible ache in your stomach because you were hungry and it was time for lunch or was it because the emotions attached to the loss of your retirement account had put all your future meals in jeopardy? Seriously, it is important to know the difference. If you are eating to stop the pain of emotionally unfinished business, you are feeding the voracious appetite of a beast that will never be satisfied! You're no longer in charge and your beast is eating you alive.

The Chinese have a saying that goes like this: "Pull the tiger's teeth before he bites." My friend and mentor and world class therapist, Dr. Ed Bryan, always said when you feel that pain in your stomach put your hand over that pain and take no action until you know where it comes from. Now, if you're following our plan and eating four to six smaller well-balanced meals per day, it is not likely you will ever unleash the beast within. Not the beast that comes from true hunger pains, that is. However, the beast of painful emotions can be a bit more complex to deal with. No one comes into this world and travels through life without facing this beast. To maintain good health and enjoy weight loss 4 life, it is imperative that we learn and implement functional methods of identifying and coping with this pain that stalks us all. In other words, "Pull the tiger's teeth before he bites"!

There are many ways of coping with this vicious painful beast within. The dysfunctional ways usually end with an IC. For instance: alcoholic, drug addict, rageaholic, food addict, etc. If you have chosen one of these methods for dealing with your beast within, it is likely that obesity is only one of your challenges in life. Again, Dr. Bryan used to say it is the "IC" that kills you. Whichever addiction you choose, whichever dysfunctional method is your medicine of choice, it will kill you in the end. It's a sobering thought! However, there is good news; you don't have to accept the counterfeit!

Choose instead to reject the dysfunctional methods of dealing with life's pains, stop and identify them, then choose a functional approach to coping with them. This is the wisdom behind Dr. Bryan's recommended course of action when he said, put your hand over the pain and take no action until you know where it comes from. Once you know where it comes from, you have begun to win the battle against the "IC."

When you make your unconscious conscious, then you can choose your course of action— dysfunction or function. Most of us can see that dysfunctional solutions are merely rabbit trails taking the scenic route to hell. A cosmic case of 'out of the frying pan into the fire.' When we attempt to use dysfunctional solutions for our problems we only accentuate and magnify problems to the point they overwhelm us. A functional solution, on the other hand, avoids the detour of addiction and sets us up for successfully confronting the pain and pulling the tiger's teeth before it bites.

This is what that might look like: Picture yourself sitting down to lunch when you're smart phone app alerts you that the market has crashed, and your once solid retirement is now merely a mirage. Do you order your favorite comfort food—times two, the strongest drink on the menu, or reach for your Xanax? All of the above or (hopefully) none of the above! Hint, any of those at this point would be a counterfeit—a false comfort. This is the perfect time to take your hand and place it over your stomach and say "there, there little one, it'll be okay," then go deep and discover the source of the pain in your stomach. In this case you won't have to be an Einstein or a Sigmund Freud to figure it out. That beast unleashed within your stomach is fear, which can hurt worse in a matter of seconds then a forty-day fast. The important thing to remember is the treatment is not the same. While food or alcohol, or name your "IC," will soothe the pain for the moment and make you feel better, at the same time it takes you way off course. It is a counterfeit solution that creates more problems than it solves. It's important that you know this. There is a solution for every problem, but finding the correct solution requires properly diagnosing the challenge you're facing. In this case, clearly food is not the answer. Alcohol is not the answer. The problem is fear. It is an emotion that is causing your pain and is also an emotion that will become your antidote.

Look with me for a minute at a new picture. You're a kind and caring parent and you have just tucked in your child for a good night's sleep. You tiptoe out of the room, find your favorite chair, and sink into it for a few minutes of relaxation with a good book. Suddenly, you're rocked from your world of relaxation by screams coming from the other room. As any parent would, you run to the room to see what is wrong. It only takes a moment for you to assess the situation and realize that it is safe and that your child has had a bad dream, a nightmare.

As a kind and nurturing parent you're ready to help your child face that fear and get back to sleep. So what do you do: (A) pour your child a stiff shot of whiskey, (B) bring him/her a dozen Krispy Kreme donuts, (C) sit and eat a pint of chocolate Haagen-Dazs with your child until he/she calms down.

Seriously, the way we treat ourselves is just this outrageous! When we misdiagnose and mistreat ourselves we can create lasting problems. Without taking you back to school to get a PhD in psychology, let me introduce you to something—a new way of thinking and a new way of using your imagination—that can equip you for success.

Let's look at that transaction again. This time, you are both the frightened child and the caring loving nurturing parent. As the frightened, helpless child, you need a kind, loving, nurturing parent to come alongside and help you face that fear until it no longer has any power over you. As the kind, nurturing parent you will do just that! You will put your arm around your child self where the pain is until it's gone, you will sit with and reassure your child self that though the fear was real it can't hurt you now. You won't offer a poison, but rather the emotion of love to counteract the emotion of fear and the understanding that there are solutions rather than simply the paralysis that fear brings with it. As a kind and nurturing parent, you have come alongside yourself as a frightened helpless child and swallowed up the emotion of fear with emotion of love and reassured yourself that solutions exist for every problem.

No, you're not becoming schizophrenic, you're just time-traveling between you as a frightened child and you as an all-powerful nurturing parent, known in the field of psychology as transactional analysis.

Remember Dr. Bryan's advice for coping with an unknown pain in our stomachs? He said to put your hand over the pain and take no action until you know where it comes from. If you follow this advice you will successfully navigate a series of transactions and play several different roles ranging from the fearful child to the nurturing parent, but most importantly, more than likely you will properly diagnose the source of the discomfort, allowing you to apply the proper treatment, which surprisingly, may contain 0 calories! A banquet table of love, understanding, and growth with no calories. Great big powerful results with itty-bitty calories, in fact none at all; isn't that what we are looking for?

The science of psychology is often just as important to weight loss as exercise physiology and diet. The vision behind this book and weight loss 4 life is a holistic comprehensive approach to wellness that offers not only weight loss 4 life, but also fitness for life, as well as emotional stability for life. To achieve the balance we all desire often requires making behavioral and lifestyle changes from a mind-body-spirit perspective. Remember, change can be a good thing, and in fact, by reading this book, you are likely ready for change, knowing that to expect different results without change is a definition of insanity.

Psychologists are experts in helping people make behavioral and lifestyle changes. By the way, you don't have to be crazy to visit a psychologist. (It's crazy people who avoid them like the plague.) If you're hitting a wall in your weight-loss-for-life journey sometimes a few visits with a psychologist will work wonders. I have found them to be as valuable a team member as physicians, dietitians, trainers, and other health care professionals.

The initial visit with a psychologist usually involves the health history and discussion about your concerns regarding weight management goals—including past efforts—stress levels, and your current life situation—including sources of support or sabotage, like friends and family. To help you, a psychologist also has to learn about your habits, your attitudes about food, eating, weight loss, and your body image. These all may or may not support your health goals.

Unhealthy belief systems that many of us express often have to do with scripts from our childhood. Did you ever hear this? "You have to eat every bite on your plate; people are starving in other countries!" (I still can't figure out how me eating all my food helped them!) There are a host of other scripts, such as, "You have to have a big dessert after every meal," or others that equate failure in previous attempts at controlling your weight with failure in life in general, which it is not. Your previous failures at weight loss do not make you a failure any more than Babe Ruth striking out more than any other baseball player made him a failure. Focus on the positive. Babe Ruth also hit more home runs than any other baseball player in his lifetime!

Managing your emotions is just as important as managing your weight. So is managing your expectations. If you expect that by reading this book something mystical and magical is going to descend in a gentle mist and cover you for a week or two and when it lifts, you will magically have that body you've always dreamed of, well, maybe you need more than just a couple of visits to a psychologist. If you understand that managing your expectations and emotions are equally as important as managing your diet and exercise, then you're well on your way to weight loss 4 life—with or without visits with a psychologist.

Please don't rule it out, though. They can be an integral part of your 'success for life' team. Tony Robbins did not get rich and famous and successful because 'psychology light' doesn't work. It does, if you want it to.

Give yourself permission to give yourself the best. What do I mean by that? Many times we do not treat ourselves as well as we treat others, which is ironic because if we do not care for ourselves, we will have nothing left to offer others. In your journey of wellness, your weight loss 4 life, do not hesitate to seek out the best experts in every field to stack the odds of success in your favor. You're worth it! Don't hesitate to find the best athletic trainers, dietitians, physicians, psychologists, and good friends who will support and not sabotage your goals.

Commit to being a lifelong learner and especially learn all you can about yourself, your physiology, your psychology, what motivates you and what doesn't, what fills you with energy and what drains the life right out of you. Take a personal inventory of what's working in your life and what is not. Make a decision to eliminate those things that are not working for you. Then carefully consider your support group. Build your own dream team for success, whether it be professionals or close trusted friends who share your vision for your life. Make a list of those things that you see are holding you back and be brutally honest. Ask your friends and professional members of your dream team to do the same. Don't get comfortable in that place of negativity and failure or you run the risk of becoming a semi-functional member of the victim class of zombies stuck in their past. That clearly is not our purpose. Our purpose is to clearly identify the hurdles in life that have held us back until now, then devise a strategy to clear those hurdles, eliminate what's been eating us, and move into a bright, successful, balanced future. Take a deep breath and remind yourself that change on purpose—with purpose—is good!

Your personal inventory of what's hot and what's not is the nucleus of your new beginning. For example, you may find that you are challenging old beliefs about food, diet, and exercise and true wellness by simply taking a look at what is working and what has been holding you back. One of the keys for positive change is becoming aware of what you are now currently unaware of. You might ask, *if I'm not aware of it, how can I be aware of it?* That's a good question. Look at it this way; if the food and wellness network were making a reality show about your life, what would you see? Oftentimes, if we step outside of our status quo—outside of the lives we lead day-to-day for a moment—and look at it as if we are watching someone else's life, we will begin to see those areas that require change!

If after watching your personal reality show you find you're not happy, may I suggest that we work on the script? How do we do that? Well, let's start by monitoring your current behaviors. Research shows that those who keep a log or daily diary of what they eat, when they eat, how they feel about it, and how they feel about the process of change, are more likely to adapt that change to fit their needs and make that change permanent. So take a look at the reality show that is your life. Begin to monitor and record your behaviors; begin to monitor and record your emotions and feelings as well. Track your activity level and record not only the nature of your activities, but also the frequency of your activities, and don't forget to eat four to six meals a day at regular intervals with smaller portions at each sitting.

Take a moment on your smart phone or on an old school 3 x 5 card to write your script as you go. Practice mindful eating. In other words, be aware of the who, what, why, when, and where you're eating. Dr. Bryan's now-famous technique for placing your hand over the pain and taking no action until you know where it's coming from is one aspect of mindful eating. Understand the things you associate with food and become aware of your habitual behaviors as they relate to your diet and exercise.

Sometimes people associate certain emotions, experiences, or daily activities with particular behaviors. For example, if you typically eat while watching TV your brain has made an association between food and TV. Here is where you may want to alter your script. You may not be hungry, but in your mind TV and eating are paired together, so when you sit down to relax and watch TV, you suddenly feel the urge to eat. You can begin to break this association by not eating while watching TV.

Watch your own reality show carefully each day and night, take notes, and review those notes. Make yourself aware of those things that you were previously unaware of, then decide which ones need to be eliminated to make a better reality show of your life and then simply change the script. Identify those times where you over-ate or chose unhealthy foods or instinctively reached for something to eat before you stopped and covered your stomach and asked, *why do I feel this way*? Is it boredom, stress, sadness? It's important to determine if you are really hungry or just responding to an emotion in a dysfunctional manner. If you are, change your script. Resist the temptation to become overly negative at the end of the day as you review your script. The purpose of reviewing your script daily is to identify and change unhealthy thoughts and behaviors. Spend more time replacing the negative behaviors in your old script with new healthy, fun, positive behaviors in tomorrow's script; after all, this is not just a reality show… it is your life.

As you already know, one of my favorite sports is tennis. I love writing that into my script every chance I get. One of the all-time great tennis players was "the Rocket," Rod Laver. Rod was one of the most gifted tennis players to ever play the game. He had great talent and expected perfection from himself. Unfortunately, that perfectionistic script, if not addressed, can actually cause failure rather than success. Fortunately, in Rod Laver's case, his father was also his tennis coach. After missing a shot that 99 percent of other human beings couldn't make anyway, Rod threw his racket in exasperation. His father stopped the show to address that script before it destroyed his son's game. He took his son's racket and said, "Rod, you can have it back as soon as you learn to hit it and forget it!" The moral of the story is regardless of how your day went, how good or how terrible your script turned out to be in this episode of the reality show that is your life, don't dwell on the mistakes or the negative; just hit it and forget it and move on. Write a new script for tomorrow that is more to your liking, more congruent with your goals, then go live it. You have creative control; you can change the script!

Since you're the producer, director, and leading actor in your play, let me share with you something that will make the reality show of your life go a little smoother. At the end of the day—after you have collected all the data, all the reviews for that day's reality show—take a moment and review the reviews like any actor, producer, or director would. Analyze the data, acknowledge the bad reviews, and embrace the good reviews, then put them aside and begin to dream of tomorrow. When you arise in the morning, it's time not for reviews, but for previews. Take five to fifteen minutes—a morning meditation if you will—and preview your day. Visualize and imagine your perfect script, then go out and live it. Start every day with a preview and end every day with a review. This keeps you in touch with the reality of your reality show as you move forward with positive anticipation of a great show tomorrow.

If you make it a practice to manage your emotions in this manner you will avoid a lot of detours in life. It is true that there are times the disappointments in life will turn to discouragement and discouragement to depression. Most of the time this process can be identified and stopped before it reaches depression, but sometimes the progression from disappointment to discouragement to depression happens with stunning rapidity. One day you may wake up and say, *Wow, I'm depressed!* This can happen to everyone. The good news is that it can be managed in a variety of different ways so that it doesn't have to become a Grand Canyon, but more like a pothole in the road of life. Potholes are annoying, but you can get around them and get on with your journey.

The symptoms of depression and weight management issues are almost always linked and the relationship is a two-way street. A study done in the Netherlands found that obesity increases the risk for depression in initially non-depressed people by 55 percent, and that depression increases the risk for obesity in initially normal weight people by 58 percent, bringing us to the age-old conundrum: which came first—the chicken or the egg? It would appear by a few percentage points that depression wins the race of which came first, but clearly the issues of depression and weight management are intricately intertwined!

Here's one reason: the part of the brain responsible for emotion, the limbic system, also controls the appetite. When this "emotional" part of the brain is disturbed, as it is with someone who is depressed, the appetite is disturbed as well, and we know if we feed that appetite without getting to the core of why we feel that gnawing pain in our stomachs, we're feeding the beast within.

Then it becomes a vicious cycle. For many people, being overweight feeds into the self-deprecating cycle of depression and it becomes a vicious cycle of, *Now I'm depressed so I'm going to eat too much of my comfort food because that makes me feel better temporarily. But now I am depressed that I'm going to get fatter the fatter and I sink even deeper into depression. The more depressed I get the more I need to eat to get rid of that vicious beast in my stomach.* You can see why it is important to apply Dr. Bryan's simple but profound test; put your hand over the pain until you can identify the cause of that pain. If it is not a hunger pain, don't feed it with food, feed it with the proper emotion.

I believe statistics show that in the care of a good therapist, talk therapy is more effective than antidepressants. Talk therapy doesn't have the side effects of antidepressants. Some of the medications used to treat depression have weight-related side effects, either causing weight loss (rarely) or weight gain (more commonly). When depression sets in, the appetite control center of the brain can get thrown off in either direction. When antidepressants are used to counteract the depression not only do they affect the emotions, but the appetite center of the brain is often affected as well.

It has been noted that the type of depressive symptoms you experience may also play a role in whether you gain or shed pounds. People with seasonal affective disorder, for instance, may often become sluggish and gain weight in the winter and lose weight in the spring, much like a bear in hibernation. While most people suffering with depression gain weight, there are those who suffer from anxiety *and* depression. It is thought that the anxiety along with depression can create an increase in metabolism, accelerating weight loss. Not the recommended way to manage your weight! How much wiser it is to manage your emotions and keep the equation simple so that you can manage your weight in an easy fashion. Untreated depression can cause weight gain, which can escalate to the point that a person becomes obese enough that it creates heart disease and diabetes; clearly, it is something to be avoided for a variety of reasons.

Because depression and weight issues are so closely linked, confronting both problems is important in order to move forward successfully. There is one magic bullet that can destroy depression and at the same time help you control your weight. You might've guessed it… it's exercise! We know that exercise increases the rate of caloric burn. We also know that exercise will decrease your appetite at the same time as it burns more calories. We saw in a previous chapter that exercise releases hormones that create a sense of well-being. Hopefully, you can see that the principles you've already learned from this book will not only serve you well in your quest for weight loss 4 life, but if the disappointment turns to discouragement and one day you wake up feeling depressed, realize those same principles will serve you well in eliminating that beast of depression from your life.

Depending on the level of depression you may need to take it slow; people often feel overwhelmed, so creating small incremental changes in the right direction is wise. Most people with depression and weight gain have reduced their amount of physical activity. This is why I spent time in a previous chapter exploring the multitude of exercise options. Oftentimes, an injury will cause you to put aside your exercise program, but if it isn't replaced with another exercise program, it sets you up for weight gain and depression. Ask me how I know. Don't forget that every bit of physical activity helps, even if it's only ten minutes here, fifteen minutes there, twenty minutes here… it all makes a difference and can serve to lift you out of your rut.

The low energy associated with depression can be suffocating, so it's best to stay vigilant in managing your emotions; however, if you do find yourself depressed, don't deepen the depression by giving up! Instead, seek help, see a qualified psychologist and together formulate a plan to alter your diet, increase your exercise and recommit to managing your emotions in a functional manner. Your physician may even need to give you an antidepressant. If so, stay in good communication with your physician as to the side effects of the antidepressant during the time you are taking it. Then work with your physician to eliminate it as soon as possible. If you notice unexplained weight gain while you are taking the antidepressant, your doctor may be able to change your medication to eliminate that side effect. It's particularly important if the weight gain is significant to also consult a qualified dietitian. You can log on to eatright.com where the Academy of Nutrition and Dietetics can direct you to someone in your area who can help.

In your personal quest for weight loss 4 life it's important to evaluate your overall health, your exercise, and what you're eating, but sometimes it's what's eating you that is sabotaging the results you want.

Now that we have made the unconscious conscious, it can't sabotage your results anymore, unless you let it. Choose to manage your emotions quickly and efficiently, and you will enjoy weight loss 4 life.

Chapter 6: The Physiology of Weight Loss

Quite a few years ago, when I was a university undergraduate student, I found that physiology was one of my favorite subjects. I realize it may not be one of your favorites and I also recall that I made a promise that you would not have to get your PhD to use the information I'm sharing with you in this book. However, when you look at the epidemic of obesity now spreading around the globe, it's clear that we need to have a better understanding of how our bodies work. In this country alone, two out of three adults are overweight. It's shocking—and it didn't used to be this way. Certainly it is wise to gain understanding about a subject that is as near and dear as ourselves. Our wellness and longevity depend on us gaining at least a basic understanding of how our bodies operate. Physiology is just that: the study of how you work. In my opinion, there is nothing more basic than knowing yourself and what makes you tick. Ignorance is not bliss and it leads to helplessness. On the other hand, the old saying "knowledge is power" is quite true. So in the interest of empowering you, let's take a closer look at you and your physiology.

Have you heard of the Krebs cycle? Hint: it

doesn't come between the wash and spin dry cycle, but it is going on inside every cell of your body at this very moment. If it weren't, you would feel worse than if you really were in your washer's spin dry cycle. Our cells are so small it is easy to take them for granted, but did you know that there are at least 800 billion more cells in your body than galaxies in the known universe? No matter how small you are, there is strength in numbers. There are approximately 37.2 trillion cells in your body and guess what? They are all operating on the Krebs cycle software program!

Remember that we learned it requires oxygen to burn that large fat molecule? So when you're exercising, if you're panting, you're not burning fat; you're burning sugar, because your body is starving for oxygen. It doesn't have enough oxygen to spare to fuel the furnace to burn the fat. It defers to the simpler fuel—the sugar burning metabolism—which can be done anaerobically (without oxygen). But you want to burn fat, don't you?

If you seriously want to focus on burning fat, an early morning workout before eating is preferable. This workout should be one where you operate in the fat burning zone with plenty of oxygen—never short of breath—so that you can carry on a normal conversation and preferably with resistance equipment or weights.

Believe it or not, if you have a typical breakfast, then walk on a treadmill or elliptical machine for an hour, and then maybe even take a 45-minute aerobics class, you might actually put on a pound or two of fat! Why? Because you're most likely burning only the simple fuel, sugar, and not fat during that time. You're operating in the anaerobic zone and burning sugar because of a high carbohydrate breakfast, so why would you gain? Well, it's all in the math. If you don't watch the math, you may find you consumed more calories than you burned in all that flurry of activity. If you really want to access the fat fuel reserves, you need to follow the directions and know your body's physiology. A ketogenic lifestyle and diet does that for you. Yes, you can eat and burn fat all the time if you want to. Just make certain to eat healthy fats and not overdo the calories. Cut out almost all carbohydrates except for certain fruits and veggies and keep your protein moderate as well.

When you exercise, make sure it is at the best time of day and distance from your last meal and make it resistance exercise without panting. The Ketogenic diet and lifestyle is used by many elite athletes, takes close monitoring, and works great for many people. It certainly is a serious consideration for those who are morbidly obese, as long as they monitor it closely and get to the gym for some engine building (resistance training, preferably weight lifting).

For people who have not built muscle throughout their lives and are obese, the first step is to begin to build muscle again! Remember, the muscle is the engine and sugar, fat, and protein are the fuels. If you want to burn fat, then you must build muscle. Fat is the preferable premium fuel for muscle to burn with twice as many calories per gram as carbohydrates and protein, and muscles love it, but first you have to have the muscles, so soup up your engine before you switch to premium fuel. Lifting weights is the best way to do that and if you do it right, you will automatically shift to burning fat. Those who try and burn the fat with aerobics classes and treadmills are likely headed for disappointment as they may only burn sugar and never get to burning fat. Remember, build muscle first; soup up your engine and you will burn fat. Nature has designed it in such a fashion that you must have a muscular body to have a lean body. That is the natural order of things.

While on the subject of fat, let me address cellulite. Cellulite is simply herniated fat cells. No cream on the market—regardless of price or promotion—is effective at getting rid of cellulite. To get rid of cellulite you must get rid of fat! The way to get rid of fat is to build and maintain a muscular body as nature designed and the muscle will burn the fat. Perhaps you'd like to get off the treadmill and stop bouncing the fat around; walk across to the gym and lift some weights. Build the muscle, burn the fat, look the way you want!

If you really want to spend time on the treadmill, I suggest that you walk a few minutes to warm up and then put it on an interval training program which will cause you to run, then walk, sprint, then walk, etc. These sprints are for a short duration and should not be causing you to huff and puff, because remember, if you're panting, you're not burning fat.

By the way, if this all sounds a little too hard for you and you're considering liposuction to get rid of your cellulite, be aware that liposuction removes the layer of fat under the surface cells, which then causes the herniated fat cells to lay up directly against muscle, which causes them to look even worse! Build your muscles, watch your diet, and with the proper nutrition and the proper type of exercise, you can eliminate your cellulite. Trust me, you will never look like a competitive bodybuilder unless you eat, drink, sleep, live, and supplement like one. You will, however, gain a more esthetically pleasing athletic body; if you lift weights and do resistance exercises, you will burn your excess fat!

If you're determined to lose fat by running, you should be aware it can be done, but it's an agonizingly slow process. If you jog or run at the level you can still carry on a normal conversation, you are in the fat burning zone, and will burn about 300 calories per hour; about half of that—150—will be fat. So, if you do five one-hour sessions per week, you have burned 750 calories of fat. At that rate in three weeks you've lost about 2500 calories. Exercise physiologists will tell you that it takes approximately twenty such sessions to lose one pound of fat. For most of us, that's enough to say it's not worth it. Are you ready to lift some weights yet? When advertised as a fat burning tool, cardio is a con. If you know your nutrition and physiology you can customize a nutrition and exercise plan that will take you where you want to go. If not, you're at the mercy of every new thing that comes along. All exercise is beneficial, for many reasons as we discovered already, but if you want to burn fat you have to follow the rules.

Scientists have determined that the light frequency our cell phones, laptops, iPads, etc., operate on disrupts melatonin function, so if you're using your device in bed be aware that it could disrupt your natural hormones and interrupt your natural sleep patterns. Why is that important? Without good sleep you will not burn the fat. Fat is very calorie dense; it is 9-10 calories/gram because of that we need a huge amount of oxygen to burn the fat. Considering that it is obvious that breathing is important as well. If you're like me, resist the temptation to hold your stomach in when you go to the gym and breathe deep from your diaphragm so that the entire lung capacity is oxygenated so that you can burn the fat by bringing more oxygen into the furnaces, those mitochondria within each cell of your muscles.

In addition to the influence of melatonin and other hormones on your metabolism, there is something called the circadian rhythm—the relationship between your body's physiology and the day and night cycle. Scientists tell us that if you work a night shift and try and sleep in the day you're going to be twice as likely to be overweight as someone who works with their natural circadian rhythm. That's not an excuse now, but if you're working the night shift, see how soon you can change that.

Dr. Udo Erasmus, author of, *Fats That Heal, Fats That Kill* and other books, has proven that good fats such as omega 3,6, and 9 assist the body in the metabolism of that fat on your hips. That's a pretty good trade; good fat makes you healthier and displaces the unsightly fat that makes you less healthy. That sounds like a deal even Donald Trump would take.

I remember watching my son compete on a stage in front of an outdoor gym in Venice Beach, California—where all the great bodybuilders at one time or another have called home—and realized one additional benefit for them lifting outdoors. And what is that? Vitamin D, which your skin produces when it's exposed to sunlight, will also help you lose weight by burning fat.

There is an old saying: you build your abs in the gym, but you reveal them in the kitchen.

The right exercises and the right nutrition will give you the results you want.

Remember that protein is essential for proper function of every physiological process in the body; vitamins and minerals are cofactors in building the right proteins that build your body. But how much protein do you need? Your body can build many of the proteins needed, so you don't have to ingest all the different proteins from your food. Athletes use this rule of thumb: approximately 1.7g of protein per kilogram of body weight works well for them.

Take a moment and look at the diagram on the following page to help you visualize our different hybrid fuels:

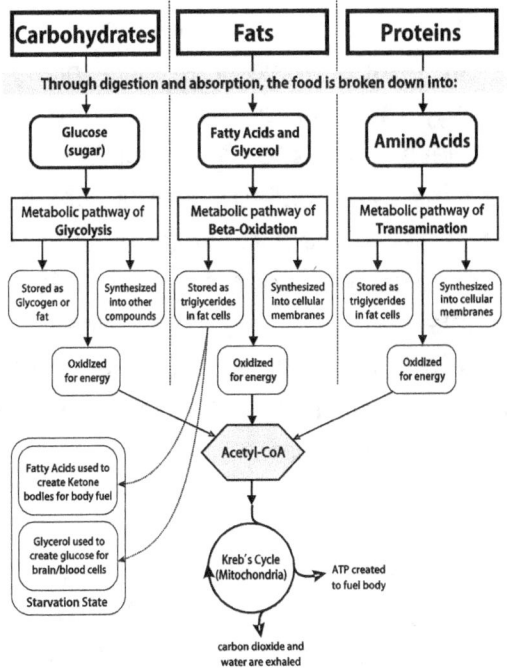

The following is a quote from a previous book I authored, titled *In Search of a Quantum God*. "The human body is a universe of its own. It is a strange at times, yet beautiful place, that leaves one in awe of the complexity that is hidden within. System after system works in perfect harmony to support human life as we know it."

Okay, let's go over the process again.

I think you will be happy to know that I'm not going to take you into the quantum physics and advanced endocrinology, biochemistry, and physiology that makes you who you are, but rather, let's just see how you digest your meals. In a so-called normal environment where food is readily available this is what happens: you eat your meal and your body immediately goes to work digesting the carbohydrates, the fats, and the proteins to make them into a form that is usable to your carbon-based life form.

The carbohydrates are broken down into glucose by various enzymes. Some are burned immediately for energy, and as the overall level of glucose in the bloodstream rises, it triggers an insulin response by the pancreas. The insulin is used to push glucose into the cells where it is made into ATP, stored as glycogen, or when present in excess amounts, the body stores it as fat droplets called triglycerides in the fat cells (adipose tissue).

The fats in your food supply are sorted out and digested in the small intestine, and then packaged into lipoproteins for various functions; you've heard of LDL and HDL, right?

Excess fat calories also wind up stored again as fat droplets in fat cells. When fats are used as an energy source, they are broken down in the cellular mitochondria through a process called beta oxidation.

The proteins in your food are broken down into individual amino acids and used in your bodies' cells to form new proteins as needed. The excess amino acids form sort of a "cachet," an amino acid reserve pool for the body to use as needed. Amino acids that are in excess of the body's needs are converted by the liver enzymes into keto acids and urea. Keto acids may be used as a source of energy, converted into glucose, or stored as fat. Urea is excreted from the body through sweat and urine.

About two to four hours after a meal, your body enters what is officially called a fasting state, when the blood glucose drops toward its normal baseline. This drop in blood sugar causes insulin levels to also decline and another hormone—glucagon—is released, which triggers the release of glycogen and fatty acids to fuel the body until the next meal arrives. During this time the carbohydrates, fats, and proteins are metabolized in separate processes into a common product called acetyl-CoA. Acetyl-CoA is a major metabolic pathway player and is an important part of the process that creates the energy molecule called ATP (Adenosine triphosphate) which powers the little engines in the cell mitochondria. I'll keep my promise; we are not going to go there, but you can explore that cycle on your own if you want. (It's called the citric acid or Krebs cycle.)

Studies show that after three to four days of fasting the stored glycogen in the liver and the muscles is exhausted, insulin levels then drop, and the body ramps up to burn its excess stored fat. Were you paying attention? Did light bulbs just go off? If it were only that simple. Let's continue. As the fatty acids flow into the bloodstream, the liver takes the excess fats and creates more ketone bodies through ketosis. The muscles continue to burn fatty acids, but decrease their use of ketones. The ketone bodies then build up in the bloodstream to a level at which the brain begins to oxidize them for fuel. As the brain uses the ketones, it needs less glucose, so the liver decreases the rate of gluconeogenesis. This helps preserve muscle tissue, as the body doesn't need to break down the amino acids to convert them into glucose. Because of this process called ketosis and the ketones that it creates the human body can survive for long periods of time without eating. HINT! It also gives you a clue of the best time and method of burning stored fat, not simply the meal you just ate.

As you can see, first thing in the morning after your night time fast (before breakfast) is when you are most likely to activate the stored fat as a fuel source with resistance training and/or interval training. Keep in mind if you are panting heavily you are not burning fat, and without breakfast you might pass out!

This has led some to develop what is called a ketogenic diet. The ketogenic diet "mimics" starvation and activates that metabolic pathway in the body. It allows certain cruciferous vegetables such as kale, cabbage, broccoli, etc. that are high in minerals and vitamins—especially potassium and fiber—and are essential, but eliminates virtually all processed carbohydrates. Protein consumption remains average, and fat consumption is boosted dramatically. Experts say it takes a diet of 70 percent fat and only 5 percent carbohydrate to activate ketosis and switch your body's fuel source from carbohydrates to fat. As you can see, that still allows about 25 percent for protein consumption that protects your muscles and the very cells of your body, which are all dependent on fatty acids and protein for rejuvenation and regeneration.

When properly implemented, the net result of a ketogenic diet protects your lean body mass and stays within healthy ranges. Essentially you switch from burning one fuel source—carbohydrate—to another fuel source that interests many of us… fat. You lose fat instead of valuable muscle mass and the best part is there are no hunger pangs, and you get the benefits of burning fat for fuel. Some of those benefits include a better HDL/LDL ratio of triglycerides, which is said to be a marker of heart health. It isn't that complicated, yet it may not be as simple as it sounds for you, so I recommend that you consult a registered dietitian or physician to guide you if you decide to switch fuel sources. I can tell you that you will be in some exclusive company if you choose to do so. Many elite athletes and elite Special Forces such as Navy SEALs use this diet for elite, peak performance, over extended periods of time.

I am certain that you can begin to see that there are methods of exercise that single out and burn fat as well as diets that single out and burn fat. Depending on the amount of fat that you desire to eliminate from your body you may choose to use one or the other or both for a short or extended period of time. My suggestion is that you make exercise and a healthy diet that you can tolerate part of your lifestyle long-term, with the option of modifying your exercise programs and diet as needed to obtain and maintain your ideal goals.

I don't think we should move on from physiology without a little chemistry as well and just a word about alkalinity. Disease flourishes in an acidic environment, and unfortunately, our modern culture promotes an acidic environment. Whether it is caused by stress or a "fast food" high carbohydrate diet or even overtraining, it is easy to slip into an acidic condition. You know that after you train your muscles get sore because of the lactic acid build-up, so even if you do everything right, you may not get the results you desire if you do not address the pH of your internal environment.

Foods/supplements like wheat grass and certain other veggies can help with that as well as adding many, many other benefits. Why not start there?

Before we do, may I suggest that you take a break, go to your local health food store or Jamba Juice and get a 2-ounce shot of wheatgrass. Why not a Starbucks instead? Well, reason number one, coffee contributes to an acidic environment inside your body. It has some other benefits such as antioxidants, and of course, a little caffeine to help you pay attention. The fact is that an overly acidic internal environment inhibits brain function as well, which could counteract the benefits of the caffeine! The neurons, which are the nerve cells that help initiate and conduct messages from the brain to the body, can descend into what is called a brain fog of forgetfulness and impaired mental acuity in an acidic environment. This state is called acidosis.

Wheatgrass, on the other hand, contributes to an alkaline environment and provides what some call organic energy. So, try the wheatgrass and if everything is still foggy go ahead and have an espresso and another shot of wheatgrass to counteract the acidity from the coffee. Then you have the best of both worlds! While it is possible to become too alkaline, it is pretty hard to do in today's society, when the diets that most of us eat create an ongoing acidic environment; and the stress, don't forget it's a contribution. Again, the key is balance in all things; we don't want you in a state of alkalosis any more than we went you in a state of acidosis.

I hear you asking, *how will I know*? Good question. You can pick up some pH test strips for urine or saliva at your local pharmacy. The best time to test is the first thing in the morning right after you wake up and before you do anything else. I hear some of you thinking this better be awfully important if I want you to test your urine pH! Well, it could be, but you can choose to test your saliva instead. There is a growing understanding among doctors and professionals in the medical field that the acid-alkaline balance is a vitally important factor in maintaining good health and that an acid-alkaline imbalance can lead to a host of diseases, including cancer.

Now that I have your attention, let me tell you what pH to look for. The scale runs 0 to 14 where 0 is very acidic. You never want to see that. And likewise, you never really want to see a 14 on your pH test strip either! Like I've said countless times in this book, balance in all things. Look for the center, something around 7.2 to 7.4, slightly on the alkaline side as your ideal. Why slightly on the alkaline side? Well, most diseases require an acidic environment, and your body seems to operate most ideally in a slightly alkaline environment. The ideal pH reading of your pH with urine test strips should be some between 6.5 and 7.5; testing your **saliva,** pH should be between 7.0 and 7.5. Notice the difference? There is a reason.

If you were to test your pH with a blood test, it should almost always come out at 7.4. Your body is a miraculous organism designed to maintain precise levels of blood sugar, hormones, pH, ad infinitum. Our organs and tissues are perfused with blood and share the blood pH of approximately 7.4; this is because of hemostasis, the body's desire to maintain that which is working, in working order. The pH in the stomach is about 3, very acidic, because of the production of the digestive acids. Everything in the stomach is then passed from our stomachs into our intestines, and is then immediately neutralized by digestive liquids and enzymes. Some say that it makes no difference what we eat. It's a point, but not an entirely valid one. Try that logic on your car or other internal combustion engine and see how it works. If you eat a balanced diet, your body receives a more balanced amount of the nutrients it needs and has an easier time keeping you "running smoothly."

As you can see, not all parts of your body operate within the same pH range. Numerous chemical and enzyme reactions occur throughout the body to regulate the pH levels. Saliva and urine have a wide range of "normal" pH values, yet health can still exist as long as these ranges are not exceeded or diminished. However, the blood pH must be maintained rather precisely for good health. One of the ways that your body maintains a precise blood pH is to draw upon its alkaline minerals stored to neutralize access acids. This is a normal process where your body borrows minerals such as calcium, potassium, and magnesium from other body tissues—such as your bones and teeth—to keep your blood pH balanced. In a chronic disease state of acidosis, this can cause a chain reaction where the minerals are not replaced into the bones at the proper levels. If that state is not reversed there can be impaired enzymatic activity, inflammation, even tissue damage and disease. It might appear that this is another one of those chicken or egg conundrums: who came first, the disease process causing the acidosis or did the acidosis cause the disease process?

Either way, it would seem intelligent of us to cooperate with our bodies' internal systems and alter our diets to assist them in reestablishing a slightly alkaline environment for good health. The less our bodies' systems have to fight to maintain homeostasis (normal environment), the more those resources can be devoted to ideal health.

Speaking of fighting, there is another field of battle that flares up when things get out of balance. Did you know that your body is a host for trillions of bacteria? Believe it or not, many of them are friendly and, in fact, your body needs them to function properly. You remember that in an earlier chapter we learned that Hippocrates, the father of modern medicine, said for us to: "Let our food be our medicine and our medicine be our food"? Well, he also said this: "All health begins in the gut." That's not too surprising today, because we have discovered that there is a microscopic war of cosmic proportions going on in there between "good" and "bad" microorganisms! Yes, your gut is a host to bacteria, yeast, and more.

Dr. Ellie Metchnikoff, a Nobel prize-winning Russian biologist, first discovered evidence of this battle between good and bad microorganisms in our digestive tract over 100 years ago. In the last couple of years new studies at Harvard Medical School and John Hopkins University have brought them into the spotlight again. Many doctors now are saying that getting the correct amount of probiotics daily is actually more important than taking a multivitamin!

Don't ask me how they measure this, but researchers in the field now say it is imperative to keep a proper ratio of about 80% to 20% in favor of the good bacteria or probiotics in your gut. If the bad bacteria tips the scales in its favor, you are likely to have a yeast overgrowth in your gut creating systemic disease and an inability to absorb the nutrients from your food. That 80% good to 20% bad ratio is the tipping point when your gut begins to start turning food into energy again. Good news: food cravings naturally begin to disappear as your body starts getting the nutrients you need to perform at your best again. An overgrowth of yeast in the gut causes you to have cravings to eat all of the food it (the yeast) wants, overriding your logical sense of what foods are healthy and good for you. We're talking about sugars, coffee, alcohols, etc.; sugar is eight times more addictive than cocaine and studies have shown that it lights up your brain in the same areas that cocaine and heroin do! So it's possible that your obesity is not because of a lack of discipline or even bad genetics or lack of exercise; it actually could be a bad yeast overgrowth in your gut! Although out-of-control gut yeast is not currently classified as a disease, it is no surprise that many health experts are now calling it the number one cause of obesity!

If you find yourself craving sugary, nutritionally empty, high carbohydrate foods and coffee and alcoholic drinks, it may not be you but your yeast demanding these foods that can damage your digestive system. That gut yeast will have what it wants… so to prevent obesity, arthritis, and numerous other diseases, it is wise to keep that healthy balance in your gut! A probiotic a day may be what actually keeps the doctor away; that is, if you choose the right probiotic.

For thirty years I've been telling my patients who have taken antibiotics to make sure that they eat a lot of yogurt and replenish the friendly bacteria in their guts. Unfortunately, most yogurts are filled with so many sweeteners and sugar that they feed the yeast instead of controlling it. That's problem number one and problem number two is related. Your probiotic must be strong enough to overcome the siren song of the sweetener or sugar that may be with it.

If you're like me you may have tried probiotics in the past to help fix an upset stomach or other digestive issues and found that they were not very helpful. The most common reason is that the probiotic was not diverse enough in the number of strains it contained or powerful enough per serving; that is, not containing enough good bacteria. Here is a good rule of thumb: look for 8 to 10 different strains and 30 million organisms per serving; then you know that your probiotic is strong enough to do some good. The right probiotic a day may be what actually keeps the doctor away.

Remember you do not have to get rid of all of the yeast in your body; you simply have to maintain a positive ratio in your favor—80% good bacteria to 20% bad bacteria—that's the tipping point. Otherwise your yeast can and will flourish and wreak havoc on your energy production, digestion, water balance, and natural fat burning mechanisms. Most people find their complexions, energy, and digestion improves, and that they are able to maintain a desirable weight with ease when a potent probiotic is working for them.

This may be one of the most important weight-loss-for-life tips you get from this book. When your system is overgrown with yeast, it can cause altered bowel functions (diarrhea and/or constipation), frequent bladder infections, thyroid dysfunction, inability to concentrate (sometimes misdiagnosed as ADHD), and the list goes on! As we've seen, the thyroid is a key player in weight control and if it can be rendered inactive by yeast overgrowth what a cascade of problems that would and does cause.

Researchers have found that the levels of serotonin are also affected by too much yeast in your digestive tract; when oppressed by an overgrowth of yeast, you may be left feeling depressed and craving more of the fuel that feeds your enemy—the yeast.

I think you can see there are numerous powerful reasons to make a probiotic—a good effective probiotic—part of your daily diet. Remember, the right probiotic a day keeps the yeast at bay…

I make it a practice to consume these daily:

2-8 ounces/day of wheatgrass juice
Recommended daily dose of Udo's oil
Dr. Wallach's 90 for life formula of essential vitamins and minerals, etc.
Dr. Sinatra's Senonol antioxidant supplement

Alkaline Body Balance drops added to water 4x/daily (Health Resources 800-471-4007)
*G-8 antioxidant drink (Pharmanex 800-487-1000)
*Immunocal Platinum antioxidant powder (888-917-7779)

    *I mix the previous two supplements together and drink them

At least 1 "Perfect Biotics" probiotic capsule (866-803-9895)

In addition, I am testing several supplements that promise to keep my internal environment alkaline, and several supplements that promise to make it easier to switch fuels to fats and make the transition to "ketosis" pain free. Stay tuned!

Chapter 7: Psychology of Success

Here's a question for you: does your psychology drive your physiology or does your physiology drive your psychology? The answer is yes.

Here's another: Are we victims or champions of our DNA? Does our DNA program us or do we program our DNA? The answer again is yes.

Our DNA makes up our genes, but is it in control? Our genes influence our intelligence, our looks, and our talents, but these qualities are not fixed at birth. If you mistakenly believe that your capabilities are derived from your DNA alone and that is your destiny, you're mistaken. Practice and perseverance and your mindset have just as much to say about your destiny as your DNA does. It's true! It is human to adopt a fixed mindset rather than a growth mindset, to live inside a comfortable box of preconceived ideas rather than live outside the box in freedom and explore your true potential, but is that the only reality? It is if you choose it to be, just as assuredly as living outside the box with a growth mindset sets the table of unlimited potential before you.

You thought you were limited by your genes.

Well, don't worry, you've been wrong before, and you're not alone. It wasn't that long ago that the entire scientific community believed Darwin, who declared our cells were empty, just filled with Jell-O-like cytoplasm. Now we know that was 'inside the box' thinking, fixed thinking based on the knowledge they had at that time. What a tremendous enlightenment the last hundred years has brought us. We discovered that rather than an empty jelly-filled donut, our cells are actually quite busy places filled with factories and assembly lines and DNA. In the year 2000 we actually managed to sequence the human genome and discovered that our bodies are built and maintained by far fewer genes than expected.

Let me share with you a quote from my last book, *In Search of a Quantum God*: "For years, the vast stretches of DNA between our 20,000 or so protein coding genes, more than 98 percent of the genetic sequence inside each of our cells was written off as junk DNA. But recently this junk DNA has been found to be crucial to the way our genome works. An international team of researchers has been working on this for a decade, but even now with these new discoveries, they say they are just beginning to touch the magnitude of the complexity in our DNA. New information, new paradigms!"

Our DNA is an elegant example of a super code. It is an error-detecting and self-correcting code that has the ability to be influenced by our environment, our diets, our thoughts, and yes, our psychology. You certainly are not a victim of your DNA unless you choose to be.

When Bill Gates remarked that our DNA is a digital code more complex than any software we have produced, it was an understatement! The super software we operate on allows us to interface with it and change it through a multitude of avenues. Keep what you like and change what you don't. You are not a victim of your DNA; rather you are the operator of the system with the ability to make changes at will. Next time you find yourself saying, "I am just no good at this," rewrite your software—just a small change at first—add one piece of code at the end of the line, "yet." Now it reads, "I am just no good at this yet." That small code correction will dramatically shift your outcome.

The next step is to identify your desired destination. Imagine what it's going to be like when you experience the outcome you desire, then begin to formulate the changes that are necessary to achieve your desired outcome. Strategize, plan step-by-step, and when you have a valid and proven strategy, visualize yourself implementing your strategies. Practice it over and over again in your imagination. What you are doing is rewriting your code! Be committed to change, plan ahead, monitor your progress, and above all, be persistent—especially when you don't feel like it. Believe in yourself even when you think you shouldn't; just know you can do it.

When I was young, my mother desperately wanted me to become a concert pianist. She was a great pianist and organist and soloist herself and spotted what she believed was the talent in me; I, however, never grasped the vision. She arranged for me to meet one of the top concert pianists in the world at that time and speak to him personally. Everybody thought he was so gifted, such a natural, but as we stood backstage he destroyed that illusion. He said, "Son, you have more talent than I do, but that won't do you any good unless you become persistent in the pursuit of your passion." Eventually I did, but to my mom's disappointment, my passion wasn't the piano.

At my father's memorial several weeks ago, an easel at the front of the church held a golf hat, a tennis racket, and a large portrait of my father. On the way to spread his ashes, as my father had requested, my mother gave me the hat and said, "Dad would want you to have this." Later I looked at it and noticed that inside the hat was a very short, poignant message conspicuously visible every time someone put it on. It said: "Love what you do and do what you love." I can tell you it is much easier to persistently pursue your passion when it is something you love to do.

Maybe you don't enjoy getting up early and going to the gym to work out every morning. But you do enjoy looking good like those who do. Your job, should you choose to accept it, is to write a new code that will connect your present circumstances to your desired outcome, and then persistently pursue your passion for the "new you." Strategize and plan to get up every morning and make that pilgrimage to the gym! Make it your passion and persistently pursue it. Do not allow anything to sidetrack you. Learn to love what you do and do what you love and you will be successful. Oh, by the way, most psychologists will tell you that love is more than simply an attractive emotion, it is a commitment. Learn to love yourself enough to do what you love and love what you do and it will see you through!

Remember the Chinese proverb I mentioned in an earlier chapter? It went like this: "Pull the tiger's teeth before he bites." It's a colorful way of saying "plan ahead"; you and I both know there's going to come a day that you do not feel like going to the gym. Well, since we both know that day is going to come, you can plan ahead and have a new script written and ready to play on that very day. Perhaps you want to use your imagination and a little role-play; like Mr. Spock, write your new code. *I do not feel like going to the gym, but that is highly illogical because my greater desire is to look like I went to the gym; therefore, I'm on my way.* In the real world I have found that feelings are real, but they're not always a safe guide to action!

I don't know about you, but another excuse that often pops up in my life goes like this: *I really don't know how to do this and I don't want to look stupid. I'm afraid I'll just mess it up, maybe even injure myself. I certainly don't want to look like a fool!* When I was younger, I never thought about the injuries, but as you can tell from previous chapters, I'm living with one now. So here's an idea for your code on that day. *I'm going to get a book written by an expert, maybe Arnold's* Atlas of Bodybuilding, *that will show me how to lift weights. I'll practice it so that I can't mess it up and I'll go light and be careful so that I will not injure myself and I will be lookin' good.* That's my personal code for that excuse …I'll loan it to you.

Here's another one that pops up now and then: *I'm so bored this morning! Going to the gym is the last thing I want to do. But I am persistently pursuing my passion even if I don't feel it, so I'll go to the gym and at least do half my workout and leave early if I have to.* I have yet to leave early! Once you start exercising and the blood starts circulating, carrying with it all those wonderful addictive endorphins that make you feel so much better, you're not likely to leave early. Go light or change up your routine, do whatever you need to do to spend your time in the gym, or on the tennis court, or any of the other exercises we explored. Just make sure you "move it, move it" and have a plan and a strategy for those excuses when they pop up. You know it is going to happen so be ready with a plan, execute your strategy, and persistently pursue your passionate destiny— the new you. Now that's quantum weight loss 4 life!

As Winston Churchill once said: "Never, never, never, give up in anything, great or small;

never give up." Sometimes when we see others who are successful in life, we think it comes naturally to them, that perhaps they're geniuses or have talent coming out of their ears. Winston Churchill had his share of failures, but they all set him up for a time when he and other leaders of the free world could not afford to fail. He became an iconic figure; he and his big cigar symbolized victory and success over extreme odds, because he persistently passionately pursued his vision.

Did you know that Albert Einstein didn't even speak and until he was nearly four-years-old? In elementary school most of his teachers thought he was lazy and would never amount to anything. I wonder if those same teachers ever really understood his theory of relativity. He never ever gave up. He used his imagination to visualize the universe and his place in it!

Consider actor and funnyman, Jim Carrey. By all accounts he had an incredibly dysfunctional childhood, having to drop out of school to help support his family when his father, a musician, failed to find work. The family ended up living in a van. But Jim Carrey never gave up and I'm thankful for that. When I see *Bruce Almighty* today, I laugh just as hard as I did the first time.

What about Richard Branson, the fourth richest person in the UK? The founder of Virgin Records, Virgin Atlantic Airlines, and now the Virgin space program. Richard is dyslexic and in his early years he literally did not know whether he was coming or going. He caught a vision of his future and persistently pursued that passion, overcoming much on his way to success. Interestingly, Steven Spielberg, Henry Winkler, Tom Cruise, Pablo Picasso, Edison, and da Vinci were/are all dyslexic as well. Now what was your excuse again? I know, I forgot mine, too.

Consider Oprah Winfrey. She was repeatedly molested by family members, gave birth at age 14 and then lost her child, all of which must've been confusing and terribly heartbreaking. She eventually ran away from home, but not from her problems. She faced them head on and overcame them as she excelled as an honors student in high school and secured a scholarship to college. Now Oprah is one of the wealthiest and most admired entrepreneurs and personalities in the world.

There will always be an excuse, and there will always be what you are wanting, what you are persistently passionately pursuing, waiting on the other side of it.

Quantum weight loss 4 life is not another diet… it's a new you!

Weight loss 4 life is much more than merely weight loss or even maintaining that weight loss for life. It's about life and having it more abundantly in every dimension, the way you know it can be. It's what you've been waiting for. So stop waiting, decide now to persistently pursue your passion… life to its fullest!

About the Author

Dr. John Luckey is a third-generation California native living and practicing dentistry in Southern California's wine country. He graduated from Loma Linda School of Dentistry in 1981. He is a father to six children—two girls and four boys—and grandpa to nine: seven boys and two girls. Besides his interest in science, John is an accomplished pilot and athlete with interests from martial arts and weight lifting to tennis and backpacking. He is actively pursuing plans to build a unique resort spa and wellness center with a mind-body-spirit approach to wellness: hwresorts.com